Spiritual Disorders

Joyless, Self-centered, Unforgiving...

By Rudolf E. Klimes, PhD, DMin, MPH

CECourses Press

Spiritual Disorders: Joyless, Self-centered, Unforgiving...

CECourses Press, 115 Kennerly Way, Folsom CA 95630

CreateSpace

Spiritual Disorders: Joyless, Self-centered, Unforgiving...

Library of Congress Cataloging Publication Data

Klimes, Rudolf Emanuel

Library of Congress Control Number:

ISBN-13:978-1481996587

1. Disorders, 2. Spiritual Disorders 3. Forgiveness

32,537 words, Times New Roman, 11 pt font.

ContED.org   ethiCE.org   CECourses.org   www.klimes.org

rudy@klimes.org

 916-984-7437

Content

This volume is dedicated to my
family, friends, and former students
who have taught me
that many of my spiritual disorders
can be overcome,
and be turned into blessings.

Preface

One evening in 1991 in Seoul, Korea, Colonel H. Britt Doze of the 121 Evacuation Hospital approached me with a request to teach a remunerated continuing education course for the alcohol counselors of the U. S. Army in Korea. I accepted. At that time, I was serving as dean of the School of Lifelong Learning of Sahmyook University and volunteer alcohol counselor for the American community in Seoul.

Many of the problems I encountered were not mental disorders but spiritual ones. Foreign army personnel, businessmen, embassy staff, and missionaries faced special problems adjusting to overseas living. Yet I found little research in that area. At that time, I defined spirituality as the relationship of a person with his soul, with his inner self and with God.

In preparation for that continuing education course, I purchased a locally available copy of the DSM-III-R (Diagnostic and Statistical Manuel of Mental Disorders). I found the sections on alcohol-induced organic mental disorders, and alcohol use very helpful.

But soon I asked myself: Why is there such a detailed manual for mental disorders available, and nothing of that kind for spiritual disorders?

Since physical and mental disorders have been around for a long time as the domains of psychiatrists, physicians, psychologists, counselors and nurses, they have been broadly researched. Spiritual disorders, on the other hand, have not been categorized in similar ways for chaplains, pastors, counselors, and health care professionals.

Following the pattern of the DSM (Diagnostic and Statistical Manuel of Mental Disorders), this volume presents eight spiritual problem areas that may be helpful in the diagnosis and treatment of spiritual disorders.

I hope that this present volume will become a welcome addition to the International Classification of Diseases (ICD), and the Diagnostic and Statistical Manuel of Mental Disorders (DSM). The new DSM-5 was approved December 1, 2012.

The purpose of this volume is to make available to chaplains, pastors, counselors, nonprofessionals, and health care professionals a manual for diagnosing spiritual disorders, based on which they can help clients.

This volume integrates spirituality with mental health, palliative care, parish nursing, and patient care.

It is also an update of Dickens's (1843) Ebenezer Scrooge, who could not find joy in London, who would not help Tiny Tim, whose money wore a hole through his pocket, who looked in vain for pleasure in work, who feared ghosts, who forgave nobody, and who kept back his workers' just wages.

From a positive perspective, some may want to call this volume a diagnostic manual for brotherly love.

1. Order and Disorder

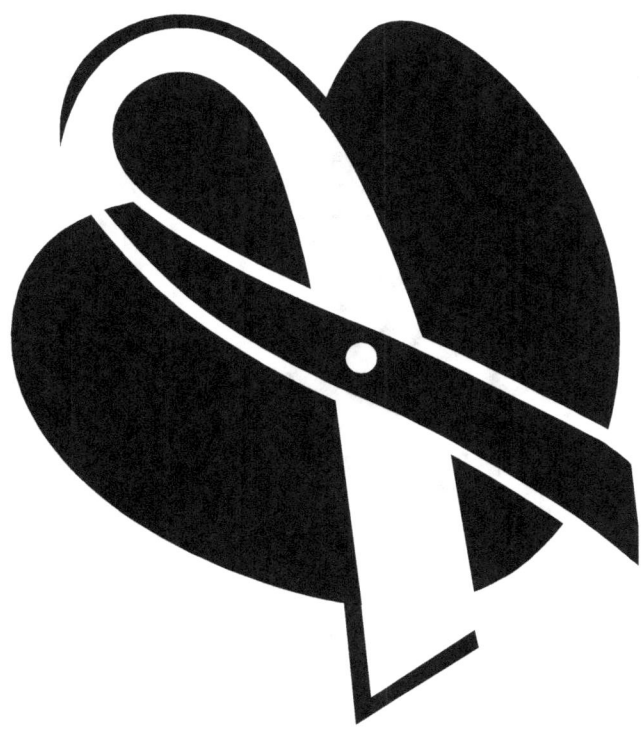

1.1 Order

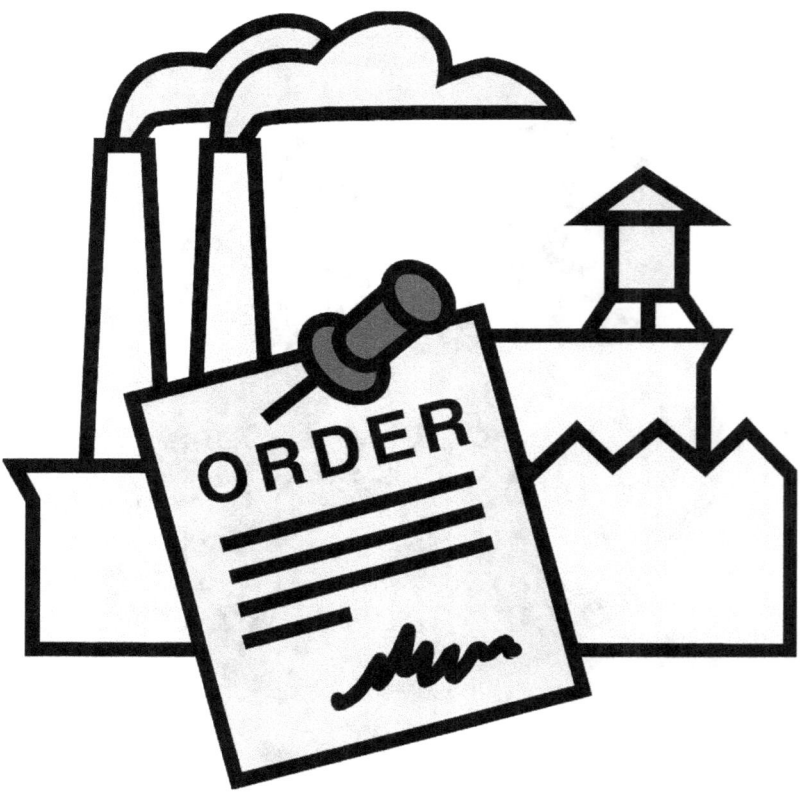

Most of us live in a generally orderly world. We set our clocks by a commonly agreed standard of time, and change them when ordered to do so in the fall and spring. We stop when the traffic light is red, and go on when it turns green.

This orderly world helps us avoid thousands of decisions, which we would have to make, if we decided to ignore the order around us. We just follow the clock and the traffic, and thus find it unnecessary to deal with these potential problems. The temperature outside, in a given locality, stays within set ranges in the summer, fall, winter, and spring. We can generally count on that and dress accordingly.

Our body temperature stays in an orderly range, so does our blood pressure and pulse. Our spiritual lives are also generally orderly. We follow our life purpose and appreciate the sun rising on another day. When things do not follow an order, many times they correct themselves. The disorder motivates us back into order.

When we lose our purpose of life, we go about looking for another one that will focus our thinking. When we lose our peace of mind, we seek a new calmness and healing for our chronic anger. Our acceptance of death can replace our fear of death. We can replace destructive values with constructive ones. We can change our trust in our achievement into a trust in a higher power. Instead of living in four dimensions (length, width, height, time), we can live in five. (add the spiritual).

We know the limits of the physical and spiritual as we are born and as we die. At these two events, the spiritual and the physical touch. In between these two events, we cannot know how physical reality touches spiritual reality. We only know that they touched in Creation, when the Spirit God made physical Adam and Eve. We are the evidence.

1.10 Visitors A an B and the Spiritual Life

Recently two unannounced visitors dropped by our house. Both had problems, and both wanted my help. Both asked me not to talk about their problem, so I limit myself here to just dealing with Visitor A and Visitor B. Both asked that I help them by praying for them, and I did. However, I was able to do more.

Visitor A described to me Problem A in some detail. I went through my list of eight spiritual disorders and easily found two severe spiritual disorders that Visitor A manifested. Knowing what I was dealing with, I could be helpful. Because of confidentiality, I will not identify the case or the spiritual disorders here.

Visitor B also talked freely about Problem B. Nevertheless, try as I would, I could not find the Problem B spiritual disorder. I went repeatedly over my list of eight spiritual disorders and all seemed in order. Visitor B was spiritually very healthy.

However, as I listened closer, I heard Visitor B complain of a physical pain that at first seemed unrelated. Then I realized that Visitor B was dealing with a stress response to a real physical problem of Visitor's B making. We started dealing with that stress.

Before we can deal with spiritual order and disorder, we have to examine what the spiritual life is all about.

While the ordinary life is material and physical, the spiritual life is the life on a higher plane above the ordinary. In some ways, we are body, mind and soul, where the body is physical, the mind mental, and the soul is spiritual.

Rabbi Micah D. Greenstein wrote that spirituality is the place where you and God meet, and what you do about it. Through it, we see the holy in everyday life. In the spiritual, we find the deeper meaning of life. Rabbi Abraham Joshua Heschel, suggested that spirituality is life lived in the continuous presence of the divine.

Spiritually healthy people live purposefully, fix the broken, help the helpless, return the lost, do what is needed, search out the meaning, collect what is precious, appreciate God's gifts, love the unlovely, and hope when all seems hopeless.

Billy Graham wrote that man has two great spiritual needs. One is for forgiveness. The other is for goodness. Spirituality involves the capacity to believe in a higher power, which gives a sense of purpose, belonging, and worth. It deals with such soul-searching questions as "Why am I here on this earth? What am I supposed to do? Where am I ultimately going?"

Simply put, we are here because we were born into this world. The Creator gave us life. We suppose to do the best with what we have. We are to love the Creator and our fellowmen now, and in the time to come. We can enjoy and follow the order around us, and be forgiven when we fall into disorder.

1.11 Using the SD1-8 (Spiritual Disorders 1-8)

The International Classification of Diseases, 9th Revision, Clinical Modification (ICD-9-CM), and the Diagnostic and Statistical Manuel of Mental Disorders IV Edition (DSM-4), are used to determine the nature, costs and time allocations associated with the treatment of physical diseases and mental disorders. They are primarily for professionals, who help in treating these diseases and disorders. Some of these deals with life and death matters. Leaving some problems untreated can result in death. There exists a medical culture that extends to about one-sixth of the USA economy.

As this is written, the DSM-IV is being surpassed by the DSM-5. There have been many questions about the approach in the DSM-4, and some of these are being corrected in the DSM-5. However, some of the fundamental questions remain, what causes mental disorders, and what affects mental disorders?

Allen Frances, MD was chair of the DSM-4 Task Force, and wrote on June 26, 2009: "The incredible recent advances in neuroscience, molecular biology, and brain imaging that have taught us so much about normal brain functioning are still not relevant to the clinical practicalities of everyday psychiatric diagnosis. The clearest evidence supporting this disappointing fact is that not even 1 biological test is ready for inclusion in the criteria sets for DSM-5." Frances, Allen. **A Warning Sign on the Road to DSM-5: Beware of Its Unintended Consequences.** (October 2009). *UBM Medica Psychiatric Times.*

We explore here the causes of spiritual disorders. Simply put, spiritual disorders are the results of the accumulation of specific wrong choices. That means, the major choices of life we make are either right or wrong. The rightness and wrongness of a choice may be determined, among others, on an ethical basic, social-acceptance basis, or a faith basis. Thus, to avoid spiritual disorders, we try to make right choices. We will deal with this more as we go along.

The SD1-8 (Spiritual Disorders 1-8) does not deal with the allocation of costs. It may deal with the allocation of time, but even that is optional. It is for both spiritual care professionals and nonprofessionals. Since nonprofessionals give much spiritual care, it is expected that nonprofessionals will take an interest in this field.

The SD1-8 usually does not deal with life and death matters. Some people do die spiritually, but many can still walk around, work, and care for their families.

For Christians, the Bible has taken the place of the SD1-8 for centuries. It describes in detail the history of spiritual disorders. The first and last chapters of that book describe a world without physical, mental, and spiritual disorders. In between these chapters are case studies of people who have struggled with spiritual and other disorders. Many of these people have moved from disorder to order.

This volume does not try to take the place of the many faith resources. It is not all-inclusive, but tries to introduce the field, and present an introductory overview of spiritual disorders. Much remains to be done, as more professionals and laypeople bring their insights and research to the topic.

So far, much of this volume is of a subjective nature. A future edition, it is hoped, will bring more objective data and evidence-based insights to the subject.

Few practitioners of spiritual care have used any systematic way in assessing the spiritual health or disorders of their clients. There does not appear to be a pressing need for diagnostics in this field. Nevertheless, as people become more aware of the impact of spiritual disorders and the possible help that practitioners can provide, the interest in this field may increase. However, since financial reimbursement is, and most likely will not be tied to a spiritual diagnosis, the field will always be more limited.

Social, situational, and environmental factors remain key considerations when dealing with client problems. The listed spiritual disorders are not in isolation, but are greatly affected by these factors, which make them easier or harder to deal with.

In the past, spiritual care had limited success. Most of it consisted of providing life order and grief relieve. Yet the needs are much greater than that. The potential of providing effective spiritual care are very great.

1.12 Spiritual Unity

In 1995, I was teaching a class for teenagers in Sacramento. Mary Whipple and her twin sister Sarah were active in that class, and showed good spiritual insights. Mary Whipple went on to join the USA Woman's rowing team as a coxswain. In the 2004 Olympics, she won a silver medal, in 2008 gold.

In 2008, Mary invited my wife Anna and me to her parents' home to view her medals and to visit. Mary put her gold medal around my neck and my friends took pictures. That was as close as I ever came to an Olympic medal.

In 2012, we watched Mary on television when she won her third Olympic honor, a gold medal. Later, as the team was interviewed, one of the rowers said that all eight rowers had to function as one body. To make that clear, one of the rowers said that they had to work as Mary's body.

To win an Olympic gold medal, the team could not afford to be disorderly. One second of disorderly rowing by one rower could cost the team the gold medal.

There was great joy in winning. All team members had worked together and none had self-centeredly dominated the team. They rowed not for the material price, but for the glory of the USA. It was hard work. However, they were at peace and rowed fearlessly the way they had planned. And they won.

1.13 Spiritual Care

Spiritual care tries to provide help and healing for those affected by spiritual disorders. In reality, it often just deals with compliance in religious matters.

Chaplains, pastors, priests, nurses, and other health care professionals probably undertake most professional spiritual care. Many professionals who provide spiritual care do not think of themselves as spiritual caregivers. Among these, there may be psychiatrists, doctors, psychologists, nurses, and social workers.

Much spiritual care is probably comfort care. Arranging the physical environment for optimal comfort removes some of the distress that comes with disorders. When in doubt, spiritual caregivers fall back on the compassionate care that expresses the love of God.

Spiritual caregivers usually do not diagnose the spiritual disorders of the people they try to help. They may work toward problem solving, but even that is usually not done in any systematic way. Spiritual caregivers are usually satisfied when clients start exhibiting some signs of spiritual life by church attendance or participation in a small group.

Since there is no accepted catalogue of spiritual disorders, caregivers give more general than specific care. This volume tries to start a dialogue about a number of spiritual disorders that are common in the general population.

1.14 The Five Dimensions of Living

The five dimensions of living, as outlined below, are built on a physical base.

1, 2. The first two dimensions of pictures, as we see them, are length and width.

3. The height of sculptures shows depth, the third dimension. All the first three dimensions present physical reality.

4. The three dimensions in a given time present the fourth dimension, or chronological reality.

5. Focusing outside of self beyond the fourth dimension is in the fifth or spiritual dimension.

Some people deny the existence of a fifth or spiritual dimension because of a negative experience with some part of organized religion. In their view, everything needs to be rational and scientific. Because of that, they deny all spiritual matters.

I see the spiritual as an equal dimension of life with the physical and the mental dimension. When people learn to step aside to focus their lives on something greater and worthwhile, they enter the spiritual dimension. Spiritual disorders describe spiritual situations that are not in their proper order.

1.15 Chaplaincy and Spiritual Categories of Intervention

Leonard Hummel and others reported the following **Spiritual Categories of Intervention** (2008) in the *Journal of Health Care Chaplaincy* (15:40-51):

1. Finding meaning or purpose

2. Enabling existential empowerment=self-management.

3. Supporting spiritual inquiry

4. Suggesting spiritual resources

5. Providing spiritual guidance

6. Promoting spiritual fellowship

7. Providing inspirational books.

It is important to differentiate between the spiritual and the religious. Spirituality is the personal quest for answers to ultimate questions about life, about meaning, and about relationship to the sacred or transcendent.

Religion is an organized system of beliefs, practices, and symbols designed to facilitate closeness to God, a higher power, or to ultimate truth, and to foster one's relationship to others in community. Religion is usually practiced in institutions.

1.16 Strength during Weakness

We are born in weakness. If someone would not look after us after birth, we could not survive. Therefore, from birth on, we live in disorder. With time, the disorder around us becomes a type of order. Nevertheless, it never leaves us.

We can never say that we are in perfect physical health or in perfect mental health. We may fall within the normal range, but there is no such thing as perfect physical or mental health on this earth.

In a similar way, we can never boast about being in perfect spiritual health. Both our spiritual strength and weakness are relative to something we cannot clearly define. We can only say that God is perfect, physically, mentally and spiritually. However, we do not come close to His perfection.

In life, we try to move from weakness to strength. We acknowledge our weaknesses, and strive for strength. However, the movement from weakness to strength is not a clear path, where we give up one to obtain the other.

We cannot comprehend perfect order, so we cannot describe it, or experience it. We can comprehend disorder, for we live in it all the time. We can describe it, and list its characteristics. Our experience of disorder seems to be not just a falling off from order, but a separate experience.

1.17 Kalish, N. (2012, June). **Evidence-based Spiritual Care: a Literature Review.** *Current Opinion Supporting Palliative Care.* 6(2):242-6.

Abstract. Purpose of Review:
"As spiritual care has increasingly been considered an integral component of a healthcare treatment plan, spiritual care practitioners have been encouraged to adopt an evidence-based orientation, just as evidence-based practice is encouraged in every other aspect of healthcare. Though the notion of evidence-based spiritual care is still developing, increasingly research is conducted in order to provide an evidence base to the practice of spiritual care. This article reviews spirituality and spiritual care literature from June 2010 to December 2011 that employ empirical research methods."

Recent Findings:
"The majority of patient-focused studies concentrate on oncology and palliative care patients. In the review period, studies of caregiver perceptions and experience came from multiple disciplines, including medicine, nursing, and chaplaincy. A discrepancy exists between the provision of spiritual care and the theoretical commitment of practitioners to offer such care. Practitioners continue to view spiritual care as part of their role to a greater extent than they provide it. This is often attributed to the absence of consensus in the field regarding the definition of spirituality, a lack of clarity of disciplinary role, and inadequate education for nurses and doctors about spiritual care. Research has further indicated that caregivers' explorations of their own spirituality correlate

with the provision of spiritual care. Although historically spiritual care has been most integrated into the care of palliative and oncology patients, researchers are developing and testing spiritual care assessment tools with other medical populations. In addition, they are evaluating these tools in diverse religious, cultural, and national contexts."

Summary:
"Conceptual analysis combined with empirical study of care giver understandings of spiritual care will assist in developing clarity and consensus about the definition of spirituality and spiritual care. Investigation and conceptualization of interdisciplinary roles and provision of spiritual care is needed for optimizing collaborative care. More knowledge is needed about how to effectively teach spiritual care."

Puchalski, C. M., Kilpatrick, S. D., McCullough, M. E., Larson, D. B., (2003, March). **A systematic review of spiritual and religious variables in Palliative Medicine, American Journal of Hospice and Palliative Care, Hospice Journal, Journal of Palliative Care, and Journal of Pain and Symptom Management**. *Palliative Support Care.* 1(1):7-13.

Abstract. Objective:
"There has been increasing recognition and acceptance of the importance of addressing existential and spiritual suffering as an important and necessary component of palliative medicine and end-of-life care in the United States. This paper seeks to empirically and systematically examine the extent to which there is an adequate scientific research base on spirituality and

its role in palliative care, in the palliative care and hospice literature."

Method:
"We sought to locate all empirical studies published in five palliative medicine/hospice journals from 1994 to 1998. The journals included American Journal of Hospice and Palliative Care, Journal of Palliative Care, Hospice Journal, Palliative Medicine, and The Journal of Pain and Symptom Management. Journal contents were searched to identify studies that included spiritual or religious measures or results."

Results:
"During the years 1994-1998, 1,117 original empirical articles were published in the five journals reviewed. Only 6.3% (70 articles) included spiritual or religious variables. This percentage, while low, was better than the 1% previously reported in an examination of studies published in Journal of the American Medical Association, The Lancet, and New England Journal of Medicine."

"While researchers in the field of palliative care have studied spiritual/religious variables more than other areas of medicine, the total percentage for studies is still a low 6.3%. To move the field of palliative medicine forward so appropriate guidelines for spiritual care can be developed, it is critical that good research be conducted upon which to base spiritual care in an evidence-based model. Recommendations are made for future studies on spiritual care in palliative medicine."

1.18 Hodge, D. R., Horvath, V. E. (2011, October). **Spiritual Needs in Health Care Settings: a Qualitative Meta-synthesis of Clients' Perspectives**. *Social Work*. 56(4):306-16.

Abstract

"Spiritual needs often emerge in the context of receiving health or behavioral health services. Yet, despite the prevalence and salience of spiritual needs in service provision, clients often report their spiritual needs are inadequately addressed. In light of research suggesting that most social workers have received minimal training in identifying spiritual needs, this study uses a qualitative meta-synthesis (N=11 studies) to identify and describe clients' perceptions of their spiritual needs in health care settings."

"The results revealed six interrelated themes:

(1) Meaning, purpose, and hope;
(2) Relationship with God;
(3) Spiritual practices:
(4) Religious obligations;
(5) Interpersonal connection; and
(6) Professional staff interactions.

The implications of the findings are discussed as they intersect social work practice and education."

1.19 Your Doctors' Spiritual Orders

If you are overweight, your doctor may order you to follow a special diet, and an exercise program. It you have high blood pressure, she will prescribe for you medication that will help lower it. Your physician tries to keep you physically well.

In a similar way, there are ways to keep spiritually well. The following seven "orders" help prevent spiritual disorders. However, just as with physical problems, one medication or diet does not fit everyone. Each person is unique, and what helps one person, may not help another one.

Part One of this volume introduces spiritual orders and disorders, Part 2 deals with the eight spiritual disorders, and Part 3 introduces ways to overcome spiritual disorders and discussion guides in ethics and faith. The objective of this book is to learn to live without spiritual disorders.

Doctors' Spiritual Order:

Be Joyous: find gladness here.
Be Altruistic: put others first.
Give: share what you have.
Serve: help where you can.
Be Peaceful: avoid stress.
Forgive: give up revenge.
Be Honest: live with integrity.

So far we have provided some context to spiritual order. Now we will examine the field of spiritual disorders.

1.2 Disorders

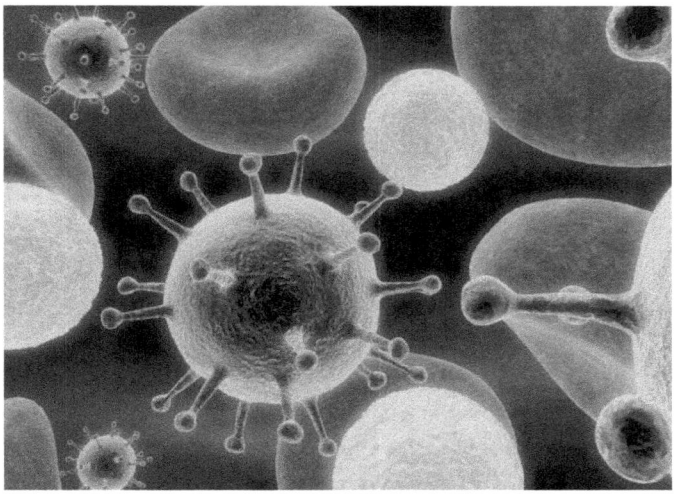

Many of our physical diseases and mental disorders affect our spiritual life, and have a spiritual impact. Spiritual disorders also affect other disorders and diseases. While the main disorders may be physical or mental, their root cause may be, in part, spiritual. People, who keep overeating, may lack a clear meaning of their life. People, who are depressed, may experience hopelessness. People, who are in constant conflict with others, may not know how to give loving service to others.

Physicians, counselors, and social workers use the categories of their professions to diagnose the disorders of their clients. In a similar way, pastors, priests, and lay workers may use the list of spiritual disorders to assist their clients.

The categories of the physical and mental disorders can be clearly defined and are thus quite specific. Many of them form the basis of payment for the healing of the disorder. The range of the specific spiritual disorders is very broad, and leaves open many forms of spiritual order. What is a spiritual order to one person may not be a spiritual order to someone else. When there is no common acceptance of spiritual order, there is then little agreement of spiritual disorders.

A case in point is the former listing of homosexuality as a mental disorder. Since that listing is currently not accepted as a disorder, it has been removed from the list of mental disorders (SDM).

The diagnosis of a spiritual disorder is just the first step in this process. Other steps include, among others, methodologies of help, planning, implementation of help, and evaluation of outcome. The 12-step program for alcoholics is usually a spiritual care activity.

The categories of spiritual order and disorder are given as continuums ranging from very good spiritual health on the left side to very harmful spiritual disorders on the right side.

 Religious or Spiritual Problem is a diagnostic category (Code V62.89) in the Diagnostic and Statistical Manual-IV Edition (APA, 1994).

We are born self-centered and many people never learn to step aside. Life demands that we learn to focus on something or someone else besides self. Most other problems are variations of self-centeredness. Materialism seeks to center life on material possessions, pleasure-seeking on pleasures.

Spiritual disorders should meet four of the characteristics below in order to be qualified as spiritual disorders:

1. Be of a temporary/passing nature.

2. Be an outgrowth of a self-centered life.

3. Negatively influence a person's spiritual life.

4. Rob the individual of deep joy and peace.

5. Relate to unethical, illegal, or harmful behavior.

Spiritual disorders are rather common and exist in various forms. Individuals may have:

1. One or more spiritual disorders

2. No significant spiritual disorders

3. Spiritual disorders that lead to death

4. Physical, mental, and spiritual disorders at the same time

5. Spiritual disorders that are outgrowths of mental disorders.

1.21 Sources of Spiritual Disorders

The four main sources in categorizing spiritual disorders are anecdotal cases, transfers from other fields, faith records, and research. It is hoped that with time, these sources will be greatly expanded and made available in book form.

At this time, anecdotal records dominate the field. While they expand knowledge, they may also be misleading and false. However, as the field of spiritual disorders is rather new, anything that helps us get a start may be useful. Future research may validate or dismiss these records.

There are related fields that may shed light on spiritual disorders. The main one is the DSM. There is a great difference between the mental and the spiritual, but some underlying issues are similar.

There is some research in the field of spiritual disorders, but it is small and not well defined. As more individuals deal with this subject, the research reports in this area will also expand and provide more clear sources for future revisions.

Like with mental disorders, we have no clear picture of the causes of spiritual disorders. As explained in other parts of this volume, most spiritual disorders are the result of wrong choices.

A woman who shoplifts at Walmart may end up in jail and in poor spiritual health (SD7). But by not stealing, the woman does not automatically avoid spiritual disorder.

1.22 Labeling of Disorders

Labeling an individual as having any disorder of any kind may be dangerous. The label itself may add to the problem.

Thus, most professionals try to avoid unnecessary labeling of individuals. Rather, they may highlight behaviors that in aggregate tend to be harmful in specific ways.

Since there are no finances or reports usually connected with spiritual disorders, there is little need for labeling. When a spiritual care professional uses labels, they are helpful mainly for her and do not have to be shared with a third party. When a student of spiritual life uses them, the labels function more as suggestions and possibilities than as facts.

People using the SD1-8 must be aware of the potential harm that they can do by misusing the categories. The use of the diagnosis must be an integral part of the treatment design.

There is a big difference between the labeling of disorders in medicine, mental health, and spiritual care. The reader must be aware of these differences and develop a labeling system that fits her environment.

Once a label is attached to an individual, it is difficult, and in some cases impossible, to reverse it. Thus, great care must be used to avoid possible harm.

1. 23 Mental vs. Spiritual Disorders

The Diagnostic and Statistical Manual of Mental Disorders-IV-TR (DSM) is the basis of identifying mental disorders. The DSM describes mental disorders as behavior that is associated with distress, disability, risk of suffering, loss of freedom, or other behavioral, psychological, or biological dysfunctions. Generally, deviant behaviors that are political, religious, sexual, or conflicts between individuals and society are not considered as mental disorders.

Thus, we may say, mental disorders are descriptions of some dysfunctional behaviors. A person may have a mental disorder when he manifests on an ongoing basis actions that fall outside the normal range of behavior.

The DSM-IV-TR forms the basis of this study. It provides the pattern by which professionals may look at both mental and spiritual disorders.

Spiritual disorders are beliefs and values that harmfully influence the direction of an individual in her daily life. They may lead to harmful behaviors. Whereas mental disorders concern physical reality, and the mental or thinking process, spiritual disorders deal with a spiritual reality and the relationship of individual to their beliefs and values. Mental disorders deal with what an individual does, spiritual disorders deal with what he or she beliefs and values. Often, spiritual disorders concern believes and values outside of our observable physical reality.

1.24 Eight Spiritual Disorders

Spirituality is a person's relationship with his soul, his inner self and with God. Religion is the institutionalized form of spirituality. Eight spiritual disorders are described here in ways similar to those used in the Diagnostic and Statistical Manuel of Mental Disorders (DSM). Each Spiritual Disorder listed here may be mild, moderate, or severe.

SD1. **Joylessness**. A form of spiritual depression that includes negativity and distress.

SD2. **Self-centeredness**. The narcissistic centering of life on self or other things besides service, and a higher power.

SD3. **Materialism**. Making possessions, money and purchasing the center of life.

SD4. **Pleasure-seeking.** Making hedonic pleasure, such as sex, sports, food, drugs an excessive focus of life.

SD5. **Fear.** The inordinate anxiety as in fear of death or loss.

SD6. **Unforgiveness.** Holding a grudge and the unwillingness or inability to renounce revenge, to forgive and to be forgiven.

SD7. **Dishonesty.** Deceptive, immoral, and offensive behaviors such as stealing, lying, adultery, and law-breaking.

SD8. **Unspecified**. Spiritual disorders that do not meet SD1-7 criteria such as unthankfulness, anger, and addiction.

1.25 Disorders as Problem Areas

There are many positive things in our lives. The positive things usually outweigh the negatives ones. People usually have enough strength to cover their weaknesses. They make sure that there is enough money in their bank account to take care of all their withdrawals. There is help in time of trouble:

a. Peace during anxiety

b. Relief during pain

d. Rest during weariness

e. Comfort during sorrow

f. Help during disaster

g. Courage during fear

h. Thanksgiving during loss.

As one truly serves one is strengthened for that service, and forgets his own ills and weaknesses. The spiritual disorders may stand alone or they may be related to physical diseases and/or mental disorders.

Some social workers have not been satisfied with the DSM approach and around 1996 developed the Person-in-Environment Classification System, or PIE. This volume has not been based on the PIE.

1.26 Nursing and Spiritual Distress

Ku Ya Lie of Fooyin University in Taiwan in 2007 developed the **Ku Spiritual Distress Scale** based on four domains, namely relationships with self, others, God and facing death.

The Hospice and Palliative Nursing Association in 2008 published a teaching sheet about the **Signs and Symptoms of Spiritual Distress.** It listed nine of them as follows:

• Questions the meaning of life

• Fear of falling asleep at night or other fears

• Anger at God/higher power

• Questioning own belief system

• Feeling a sense of emptiness; loss of direction

• Talking about feelings of being left by God/higher power

• Seeking spiritual help

• Questioning the meaning of suffering

• Pain and other physical symptoms, that can be expressions of spiritual distress as well.

1.27 Severity of Disorder

Like in the DSM, spiritual disorders may be classified as mild, moderate, severe, and in remission. The symptoms must be evidenced over time, usually for three months or more.

In mild disorders, the number of negative symptoms observed is the minimum or close to minimum required to make a diagnosis at the stated time. For example, if four out of eight symptoms are required to make a diagnosis of a disorder, only four or possibly five symptoms were observed.

Moderate disorders are those that fall between mild and severe, and produce observable impairments.

Severe disorders are those where the number of symptoms is clearly in excess of the minimum or middle number of the symptoms required. For example, if three symptoms are required, six or more symptoms are observed.

A disorder is in remission when there is evidence that the individual had in the past a mild, moderate or severe spiritual disorder, but that at the present time none of the symptoms warrant a diagnosis of the disorder. When no symptoms of the disorder remain, it is called full remission.

There are some groups of people with severe spiritual disorders, where leaders of dangerous cults are so persuasive and evil, that members are willing to die with them, to kill others, to give them their all, or to have sex with them.

1.3 Service

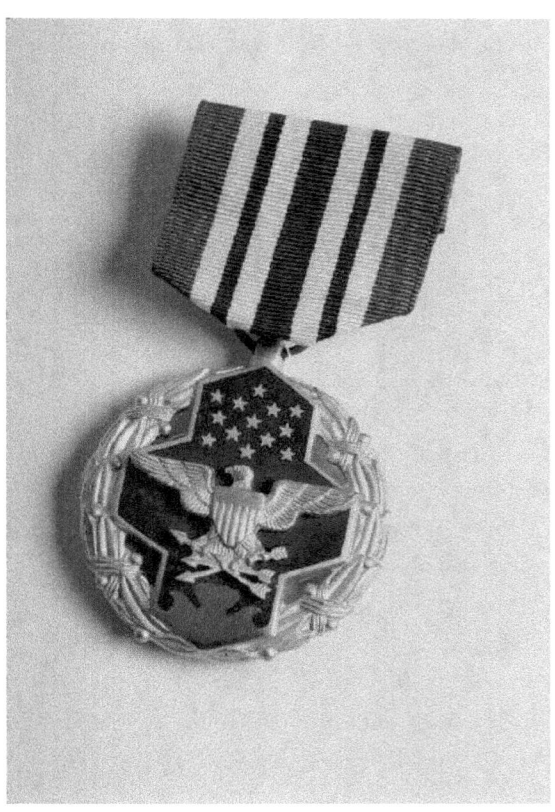

Many people feel that they should serve and help. They focus on serving others who may be in need. Service to many does not include self-service, where the ego is the center of the universe.

Service can be selfish or unselfish. In selfish service, we make our reward central and highlight whatever we can get out of service. Selfish service really does not help others, but it feeds the ego, to make the server feel better.

When we serve unselfishly, we do not focus on what we do, but how we help someone else. When we serve someone else unselfishly, we forget ourselves and do all to make life better for our friend.

All people have some beliefs and some value systems. They may deny the existence of the supernatural or value strange priorities, but they believe and value.

Spiritual life is usually associated with religious expressions, but it goes way beyond organized religion, churches, sacred scriptures, or prayer. The most common spiritual disorder is self-centeredness that excludes others from a person's life. There are people who show little formal spiritual concern that are spiritually healthy.

We do not claim to validate the eight categories on scientific grounds. The categories have risen out of research and the 60-year experience of the author in teaching, pastoring, and administering institutions where the spiritual life was important. Readers need to strive continually for an ethical use of these categories.

There is a great need to test the reliability of the categories. The author invites all qualified individuals to assist in this and make these studies available for the second edition.

1.31 Do No Harm

Order tends to bring help disorder tends to foster harm. Actually, disorder, be it physical, mental or spiritual, nearly always brings harm. Thus, we try to stop or reduce disorders as much as possible.

There are two types of disorders, namely those we can do nothing or little about, and those we can avoid. Most spiritual disorders are of the later type and thus can be avoided by better choices.

People seldom think through the full consequences of their choices. Good choices usually have good consequences bad choices have bad consequences. Nevertheless, there are times, when good choices have bad consequences. My young friend Michael joined the armed services, a good choice. In Afghanistan, one of his close friends was killed and he misses him, a bad consequence.

We try to avoid harm, but not at any cost. We have to be true to ourselves. We may accept the loss of something, in order to help in something else. We may give up our wisdom teeth in order to avoid tooth decay.

Do no harm to others or to self. There are some who will avoid all harm to others, but who readily harm themselves. Actually, when a person harms himself, he also harms others. People around you care and are negatively affected when you harm yourself.

1.32 Morality

Morality deals with the principle of right and wrong in human conduct. Because spiritual disorders are results of wrong choices, morality plays an important part in spiritual disorders.

A person with many spiritual disorders may lack a good moral character. On the other hand, he may be struggling with many issues that affect his morality. That struggle may be an honest struggle and desire to do right, or it may be a pretext for doing wrong.

An example of a moral code is the Golden Rule that states that, "One should treat others, as one would like others, to treat oneself." That type of behavior is good and moral; the opposite is evil and immoral.

Morality is the answer to the question 'how ought we to live' on the individual level. Most people try to live helpfully, but some go on living harmfully. People often become conscientious of their disorders and try to find healing for them.

All crimes are immoral acts, and are thus harmful. So are illegal acts and unethical acts. Society tries to teach morality through its emphasis on the family, education, and religion. Where these institutions are weak, immorality flourishes.

1.33 Relational Spiritual Disorder

In considering spiritual disorders, one must examine the circumstances under which the disorder expresses itself. At times, that may be very important, and at other times, that may be unimportant.

Spiritual disorders are often relational. They may apply only to one person, to one or more groups, to all persons, or to a higher power. It is possible to have a specific spiritual disorder in relationship to one person, but not have that disorder in relationship to other individuals, groups, to all persons, or to God. There are people who fight constantly with their spouses, and live in perfect peace with their neighbors or fellow workers.

However, while applying to the relationship of only one person, spiritual disorders may be nevertheless important, troublesome, and severe. Thus, they may need to be dealt with.

In that case, spiritual disorders are similar to mental disorders, which require a careful examination of circumstances. At times, spiritual disorders may be more in the relationship itself than in the individual diagnoses. So far, little is known about this topic.

The categories of spiritual disorder do not apply to people who may not be able to tell right from wrong, that is children under the age of seven, the insane, and the demented.

1.34 Northridge, W. L. (1961). **Disorders of the Emotional and Spiritual Life,** Great Neck, NY: Channel Press.

Dr. Northridge, a psychiatrist, produced one of the earliest useful books on spiritual disorders. He carefully developed 14 areas, and discussed them in detail. Dr. Northridge focused heavily on what we now call Spiritual Disorder 6 (SD6), some on SD8, and not at all on SD3 and SD4. The areas (chapter titles of the Northridge book) that the present author developed further are as follows:

SD1. Joylessness. Depression, the Martyr Complex, Stress, Grief, and Sorrow.

SD2. Self-centeredness. The Malady of Pride.

SD3. Materialism.

SD4. Pleasure-seeking.

SD5. Fear. Fear of Old Age and Death.

SD6. Unforgiveness. Healing through Forgiveness, The Unpardonable Sin, The Overanxious Mind, Our Resentment and our Health, In Search of Scapegoats.

SD7. Dishonesty.

SD8. Unspecified. Morbid Doubt, Jealous Moods, Prejudice, unthankfulness.

1.35 Spiritual Transitions

Small children usually follow the spiritual teachings of their parents and teachers. If their parents or teachers are not spiritually active, the children will most likely also be inactive. To some, it is beautiful to hear small children sing praises to God, to enjoy Bible stories and to help their siblings with their tasks.

There seem to be at least four transition ages when people step from one spiritual environment into the next one. The exact age may vary, but the four transition age-ranges are the often rebellious teen-ages years, the midlife crisis of the 40s, the retirement adjustments of the 60s, and health challenges of the 80s.

The teen-age years are one of first big tests of most children. About half of the children who have a very normal and healthy spiritual life as children are not able to transfer it into the early 20s. As children, they are very comfortable in the spiritual environment around them and seem to enjoy it. They do not manifest any unusual spiritual disorders. Many of them are sheltered from the big problems of life.

The children who rely only on the social support and values of others usually cannot make the transition into spiritual adulthood. Their spirituality has to be their own. Their family religion has to become their personal faith. They can develop their own faith by their own deep participation in spiritual issues. Teenagers who do not anchor their souls on some certainties are swept away by the developing confusion around them.

Of the four spiritual transitions, the teenage one is the most difficult. Boys seem to have a harder time with it than girls do. The healthy spiritual development of youth seems to be so easily snuffed out by a powerful spiritual disorder. Each new generation brings its own problems into its culture. What helped the 60-year one long ago seems irrelevant to today's teenager.

The midlife crisis of the 40's is usually connected with a realization that one's great dreams will not be realized. It often is a downgrading of expectations, including spiritual expectations.

Then you come to your 60's and 80's. These ages involve much loss and giving up. However, a loss in one area can be a gain in others. The strength of youth can give place to the joy of maturity. By then, you have usually sifted out what is important and what is not. You may be willing to drop the unimportant and focus on the important.

The four spiritual transitions either take you up to spiritual maturity and strength, or wash you out and leave you with a weaker spiritual life. These transition points are opportunities for growth and healing. They make you realize that you do not stay the same all your life. New spiritual disorders may be a harbinger of trouble to come. That is why the study of spiritual disorders is so important.

2. Spiritual Disorders

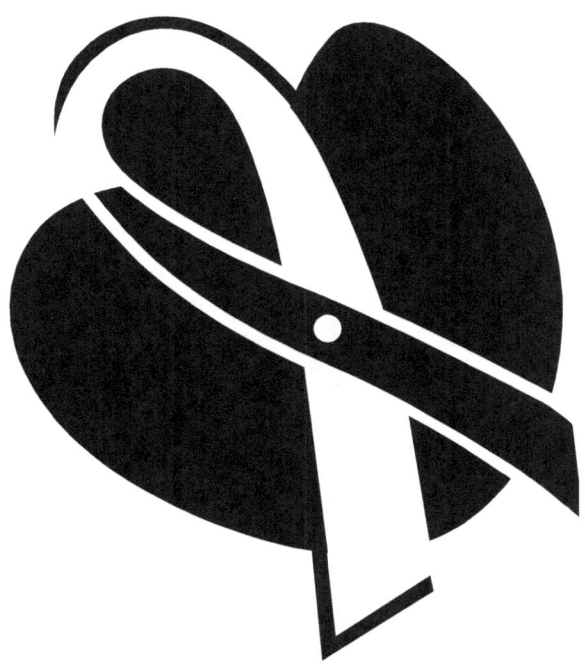

Health professionals often claim to deal with the whole person, which includes body, mind, and soul. The body is the physiological-biological dimension that is observed with our five senses. The mind works mainly through thinking. The soul is in the spiritual area of life. These three are closely connected, and affect each other. Whatever touches the body, usually also touches the mind and soul.

In this section, the author suggests eight Spiritual Disorders that may form the basis of spiritual diagnosis and treatment. The presentation follows the pattern set in the Diagnostic and Statistical Manual of Mental Disorders (DSM). The below eight Spiritual Disorders are based, in part, on research and the experience of various groups of health care professionals and clients.

2.1 Joylessness Disorder

2.2 Self-centeredness Disorder

2.3 Materialistic Disorder

2.4 Pleasure-seeking Disorder

2.5 Fear Disorder

2.6 Unforgiveness Disorder

2.7 Dishonesty Disorder

2.8 Unspecified Disorder

2.1 Joylessness Disorder

SD1

2.11 Spiritual Joylessness Disorder

A habitual manifestation of depressed moods that is characterized by skepticism, resistance, refusals, opposition, denial, negation, counteraction, contradiction, and a definite lack of joy, optimism, affirmation, courage, positivity, and drive as manifested by at least four of the following:

a. finds no joy in personal relationships

b. lacks the ability to enjoy spiritual blessings

c. appears constantly overly serious

d. does not comprehend the joy beyond the immediate

e. expresses long-term discouragement

f. refuses to explore areas that may bring joy

g. sees great difficulties in everything undertaken

h. manifests extensive pessimism.

There are different types of joy. A widow may look back and miss her time of married bliss. But as she serves others, she may learn that each stage of life provides its own great joys and blessings.

2.12 Characteristics of Joylessness Disorder

Associated Features and Coexisting Disorders

Whereas 296.2x - 296.3x depression in the DSM-IV-TR is a mental disorder, joylessness is a spiritual disorder. The two may be related but often they are not in the same area. Joylessness is often associated with negativistic behavior.

Onset Age and History

Joylessness usually starts in the teenage years, when children start questioning many issues and find no pleasure in the areas where they should find satisfaction. Sports seem more important than church. Joylessness may also be part of the middle-age crisis that besets individuals in their 40s. In some individuals, it may develop around the early 60s when they lose interest in learning, work, fellowship, and church.

Impairment in Social and occupations functions

Joylessness impairs social functioning in that joyless people bring very little to relationships.

Prevalence Range

Spiritual joylessness is very likely the most common spiritual disorder. Periods of mild joylessness may touch a majority of people. Joy itself is a healing agent for many spiritual disorders. Some spiritual joylessness may not appear very spiritual, but it interferes with healthy living.

2.13 Joyless Jane

Jane grew up in a good home and enjoyed life. She did well in school and college. Upon graduation, she took a job as an elementary teacher in the local public school. She was good at keeping her friends. She would get together with her college graduation classmates every year and really enjoy them.

Her three great areas of joy were her work, her family, and her friends. Soon, all this ended. In her early 30s, Jane met her husband-to-be, got married, had two children in three years, and moved from the west coast to the east coast.

After marriage, she never went back to work outside her home. She was far away from her family and, while they kept in touch, Jane was out of sight, and out of mind. She exchanged some email with two of her friends, but she did not have the money to get together. Her life, while busy, had become joyless. She missed her elementary school children, family, and friends. Her areas of joy had collapsed.

Her choices now were:

____ Try to resurrect her former life support, get a job, and reconnect with her family and friends.

____ Try to find new areas of joy like a church, reading, camping, or neighborhood groups.

____ Build on her past areas of joy, volunteer with children, make new friends, and save up for an annual trip home.

2.14 Bekelman, David. B., Sydney, M., Dy, M. Diane M. Becker, Wittstein, Ilan S., Hendricks, Danetta E., Yamashita, Traci E., Gottlieb Sheldon H. (2007, April). **Spiritual Well-Being and Depression in Patients with Heart Failure.** *J Gen Intern Med. 22(4): 470–477.*

"Spiritual well-being is associated with less depression in patients with terminal cancer, but this relationship has not been studied in patients with heart failure. Spirituality may play a major role in functioning, health status, and quality of life in heart failure patients; because spiritual concerns are important to them and are significant in how they view and cope with their illness."

"Spirituality is often equated with religious faith; however, a broader and more inclusive definition is 'the way in which people understand their lives in view of their ultimate meaning and value.' Spiritual well-being refers to one's spiritual state of affairs. This conceptualization of spirituality is emphasized in palliative care, which has been advocated in patients with heart failure to relieve suffering and distress."

"The primary objective of this study was to identify the relationship between spiritual well-being and depression in an elderly heart failure population in the context of other common risk factors for depression. Greater spiritual well-being, particularly meaning/peace, was strongly associated with less depression."

2.15 Monod, Stefanie, Etienne Rochat, Christophe J Büla, Guy Jobin, Estelle Martin, and Brenda Spencer. (2010). **The spiritual distress assessment tool: an instrument to assess spiritual distress in hospitalized elderly persons.** *BMC Geriatr.* 10: 88.

"Although spirituality is usually considered a positive resource for coping with illness, spiritual distress may have a negative influence on health outcomes. Tools are needed to identify spiritual distress in clinical practice."

"A three-step process was used to develop the Spiritual Distress Assessment Tool (SDAT): 1) Conceptualization by a multidisciplinary group of a model to define the different dimensions characterizing a patient's spirituality and their corresponding needs; 2) Operationalisation of the Spiritual Needs Model within geriatric hospital care leading to a set of questions; 3) Qualitative assessment of the instrument's acceptability and face validity in hospital chaplains."

"Four dimensions of spirituality (Meaning, Transcendence, Values, and Psychosocial Identity) and their corresponding needs were defined. A formalized assessment procedure to both identify and subsequently score unmet spiritual needs and spiritual distress was developed."

"The SDAT appears to be a clinically acceptable instrument to assess spiritual distress in elderly hospitalized persons."

2.16. Maselko, J, S., Gilman, E., and Buka, S. (2009, June) **Religious service attendance and spiritual well-being are differentially associated with risk of major depression.** *Psychol Med.* 39(6): 1009–1017.

"The study investigated the independent influence of religious service attendance and two dimensions of spiritual well-being (religious and existential) on the lifetime risk of major depression. Data came from the New England Family Study (NEFS) cohort (n=918, mean age=39 years). Depression according to DSM-IV criteria was ascertained using structured diagnostic interviews. Odds ratios (ORs) for the associations between high, medium and low tertiles of spiritual well-being and for religious service attendance and the lifetime risk of depression were estimated using multiple logistic regression."

"Religious service attendance was associated with 30% lower odds of depression. In addition, individuals in the top quartile of existential well-being had a 70% lower odds of depression compared to individuals in the bottom quartile. Contrary to our original hypotheses, however, higher levels of religious well-being were associated with 1.5 times higher odds of depression. Religious and existential well-being may be differentially associated with likelihood of depression. Given the complex interactions between religiosity and spirituality dimensions in relation to risk of major depression, the reliance on a single domain measure of religiosity or spirituality (e.g. religious service attendance) in research or clinical settings is discouraged."

2.17 Joylessness, Depression and Suicide

Normally, we live by hope. When hope dies, depression sets in. Depression is a mental disorder, but some of it has spiritual overtones. Depression, or as we call it hear joylessness, can also be a spiritual disorder that is similar to the mental disorder. Any type of depression can lead to suicide.

There is a complete mental health and behavioral health profession, that is charged with the prevention of suicide. That includes psychiatrists, social workers and behavioral health nurses. That group has not been very effective in preventing suicide, even of soldiers who are actively seeking help.

Individuals need to experience the positive joy of living to overcome the discouragements that life brings. Without that spiritual joy, depression is often too strong to keep going.

In some cases, suicide is a self-centered spiritual disorder where the presence of God and of family and others does not seem to matter and help. At times, the fear of the coming problems is too great to be overcome by the joy of living. In suicide, people often deceive themselves to think that death is putting an end to the problem, when in actuality; it creates a whole train of problems in its wake.

Spiritual help is more that a mental health exercise. It introduces individuals to a dimension that goes clearly beyond the physical and mental, to that which is outside of our power. It anchors the soul on something greater than self.

2.2 Self-centered Disorder

SD2

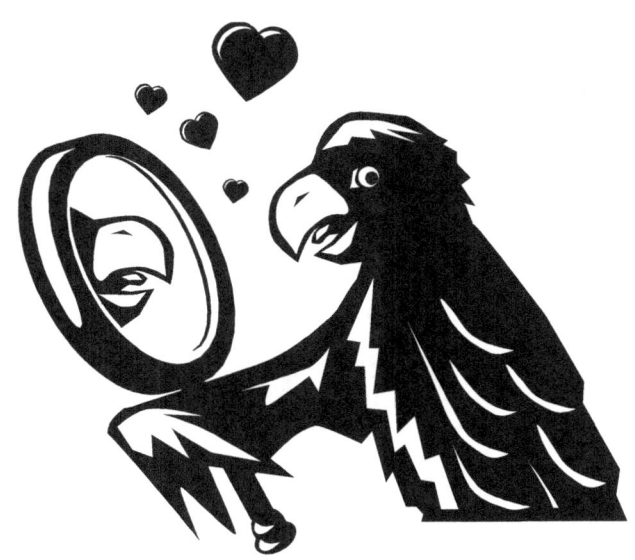

2.21 Spiritual Self-centered Disorder

A controlling pattern of excessive love of self, and the inability to give others or other things their due place in their lives, as manifested by at least four of the following:

a. takes on tasks that feature her great power

b. neglects to delegate tasks to other able team members

c. works to achieve her self-advancing goals

d. manifests an excessive amount of self-importance

e. feels entitled to special considerations

f. does not feel the pain of others

g. is uncomfortable with submitting to others

h. lives in a fantasy world of unrealistic greatness.

Narcissism as a psychological disorder sometimes stands alone, but it is often associated with the spiritual self-centered disorder. While related, the two are not the same.

2.22 Characteristics of Self-centered Disorders

Associated Features and Coexisting Disorders

People with self-centered disorder are often troubled when their grandiose plans go unrealized. They may over-emphasize clothing, successes, or youthfulness. Feelings may be faked in order to appear popular.

Onset Age and History

Babies are born self-centered. Their main concern in life is the obtaining of food and comfort. They cry for food when hungry and for comfort when they are wet or in any way uncomfortable. As they grow into childhood, most of them learn to cope with delays and difficulties. In their teens, most learn that they are not the center of the universe and may have trouble submitting to the social order around them.

Impairment in Social and Occupations Functions

People in positions of power have many opportunities to develop self-centered disorders. Their world focuses on things they control. They are tempted to control too much.

Prevalence Range

This disorder is very common and generally accepted. There is very little prohibition against it. It is more common in men than women, and remains one of the greatest hindrances to spiritual growth.

2.23 Self-centered Sam

Sam filled the room wherever he went. Just looking at him made you realize that he was important. He constantly kept using the I-word and would often refer to his high position and title. Sam was Sam-centered.

There was no room left for others beside Sam. Even when he talked of serving others and God, that service seemed secondary. To most, Sam's self-centeredness did not seem offensive. He wove it in so naturally, that it looked like he was born a superior being. He was very unaware that his ego was constantly oozing out of him.

Sam has a very hard time recognizing how others feel about issues, on which he is to work with someone else. He is not able to serve unselfishly, and to put himself as last in the line. Sam has to be first in everything, even if that is only in his imagination. He often takes advantage of others in order to achieve his egotistical ends.

How can you help Sam? Which way would be best?

___ Help Sam recognize his limitations. Once he realizes that he is not quite so special, he may appreciate the contributions of others, and the help of God.

___ Suggest that Sam join an open group, where people can honestly share their strengths and weaknesses.

___ Work with Sam to help a person in real need.

2.24 Pride

It is important that we all respect ourselves and look after ourselves. However, when we center our lives on self and become egocentric and proud, we get into trouble.

It is quite easy and natural to be self-centered. It makes us feel good and respected, even when there are no good reasons to feel good and respected. We make ourselves the judge of our worth and ignore everyone else who may have an opinion on our value. We become critical of others and blind to our own weaknesses. We lose a grip on the reality around us.

The self-centered person has a false sense of pride. He is conceited and has an overly high opinion of himself. Pride has been listed as the first of the seven cardinal sins. A prideful person esteems himself higher than he should, for he is not as great as he thinks he is.

The opposite of pride is humility. Whereas pride is a spiritual disorder, humility is broadly considered a good characteristic. Pride cuts off relationships; humility opens them. Pride focuses on self, humility focuses on service to others. Pride shows your real poverty, while humility may show our real riches of character.

There is also a healthy pride that is in no way self-centered. We may take proper pleasure and satisfaction in our work and achievements. A marine can take pride in his faithful service to his country. A father may be proud of his son. There is nothing wrong with that.

The self-centered person strives for honor mainly for himself. For him, others and God do not seem so important. On the other hand, a healthy spiritual person will first seek the honor of God, then of others whom he serves, and lastly for himself.

To be spiritually healthy, we should focus our love on others, not on self. When we love only ourselves, we ignore the God who is much more worthy of our love. When we love God, we step aside from our self-centeredness, and all parts of our lives take their proper place. When we mainly love ourselves, we take on an excessive burden to protect ourselves at all costs.

In most cases, the love of self is not real love. In love, we wish the best for others and work for it. It is quite natural to want the best for yourself. However, when we do so at the expense of others, we do not express love. We manifest self-centeredness.

We keep God and others in our lives, so that we can relate to them, and serve them. We lose that relationship when we are self-centered and proud. We can ignore God and others, but at a cost. When self takes the main place in people's lives, God and others are pushed to the side. Our selves are not steady and helpful enough to take the central place in our lives. We need a higher power and a clear focus.

2.25 Spiritual Life and Death

When a person's life is centered on serving others and God, there is a vibrancy to it that permeates a person's whole physical and mental being. It provides other-centeredness that is healthy and enriching.

When on the other hand, self-centeredness takes over; there is a limiting of spirituality and sometimes a death of spiritual life. Self is an unsuitable leader of the spiritual life. Self is limiting and any expansion of it just illusionary. We may think we are great, but compared with others and God, we have very little to offer.

There are people walking about that are spiritually dead. They are insensitive to the needs of others and God. They do not appreciate others and God. They live only on a physical and mental plane.

In a similar way, materialism, pleasure-seeking, fear, unforgiveness and dishonesty can limit and choke spiritual life. There is no room for the spiritual in an exclusively material, pleasure-seeking, fearful, unforgiving and dishonest world. Disorder takes over completely and crowds out those aspects of life that make the soul sing and grow.

It is unusual to bring a spiritually dead person back to life. But it happens. It may be our responsibility to recognize the danger signals of spiritual disorders, and to find early healing.

2.26 Föller-Mancini, Axel, Heusser Peter, Büssing, Arndt, (2010). **Self-centeredness in Adolescents: An empirical study of students of Steiner schools, Christian academic high schools, and public schools.** *Research on Steiner Education,* Vol 1 No 2.

Abstract. "We intended to further analyze the attitudes of 17 year old high school students associated with more self-centered positions on the one hand and altruistic tendencies on the other hand. Previous findings indicated that `self-centeredness´ is particularly valued by boys while less so by girls. In a sample of 521 German high school students (mean age 16.6 ± 0.70 years) recruited from Christian schools (38%), Waldorf schools (36%), and public (state-funded) schools (27%), we investigated influencing factors such as schooling, individual ideals / ethics, and spirituality. We confirmed that `self-centeredness´ was expressed significantly lower in female than in male students; yet there were no significant differences which could be ascribed to the different school types. Regression analyses indicated that this self-centered position can be predicted best (R^2 = .211) by an attitude focusing on one's own well-being and the conviction that pity for others prevents them from taking the initiative themselves; these predictors are negatively modulated by satisfaction with the school situation, a spiritual Quest orientation, and the ideal of helping others. Although the school type by itself is not a significant predictor of the respective attitudes, the associations between self-centeredness and ethical ideals nevertheless differed between students of the different schools types."

2.27 The Empty Self

Moreland, J.P. (1997). **Love your God with all your mind: The role of reason in the life of the soul**.: *Colorado Springs, CO.: Navpress Publishing Co.*

Moreland (1997) identifies seven attributes of what psychologists call the "empty self," which has been growing in "epidemic proportions" in America (p. 88). "The empty self is constituted by a set of values, motives, and habits of thought, feeling, and behavior that perverts and eliminates the life of the mind and makes maturation in the way of Christ extremely difficult. There are several traits of the empty self that undermine intellectual growth and spiritual development." (p. 88). Some of the traits are self-interest, self-infatuation, self-as-exterior, passivity, and self-fatigue.

"The narcissist evaluates the local church, the right books to read, and the other religious practices worthy of his or her time on the basis of how they will further his or her own agenda.... Narcissists see education solely as a means to enhance their own careers. The humanities and general education that historically were part of a university curriculum to help people with the intellectual and moral virtues necessary for life directed at the common good just do not fit into the narcissist's plans. As Christopher Lasch notes, '[Narcissistic] students object to the introduction of requirements in general education because the work demands too much of them and seldom leads to lucrative employment'" (p. 90).

2.28 Chang, Maria Hsia. (2009). **Pathological Narcissism, A Spiritual Disorder**. Professor, Political Science, University of Nevada, Reno..
<http://abusesanctuary.blogspot.com/2007/02/pathological-narcissism-spiritual.html>

"The spiritual narcissist. these are those who ooze with false piety, having a false conception of themselves as supremely virtuous."

"A fifth-century theologian who called himself Dionysius the Aereopagite once wrote in The Divine Names that, 'The denial of the true self is a declension from Truth.' In the last analysis, in constructing and clinging to their false selves, the entire persona of the Narcissist Personality Disorder (NPD) is a big lie. That being so, I have come to believe that NPD is not a psychological disorder at all, but a moral and spiritual disorder. An intrinsic attribute of the NPD syndrome is deception- of oneself and of others- in the service of maintaining the grandiose false self. Philosopher Rene Descartes wrote that 'willful deception evidences maliciousness and weakness.' A person does not deceive without thinking about it and willing it. One does not lie unless one intends to hide the truth, which means that one knows that one is being deceptive. Nor can the NPD put together and maintain the elaborate and intrinsic NPD syndrome of attitudes (e.g. using others for self-aggrandizement, attractive social mask, secrecy, evasion, lying, scape-goating etc.) without conscious effort."

2.3 Materialistic Disorder

SD3

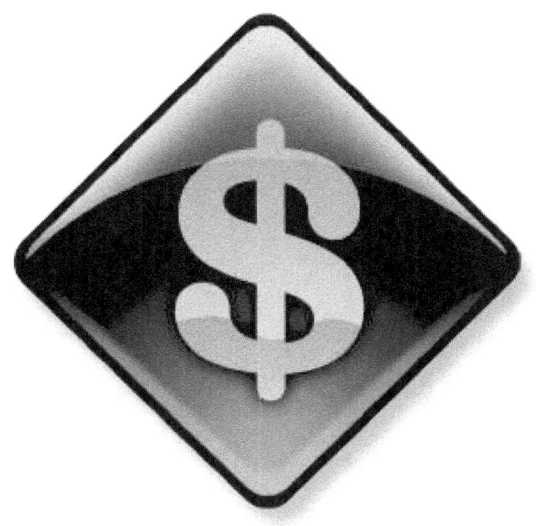

2.31 Spiritual Materialistic Disorder

A pattern of behavior that focuses on obtaining and keeping money, investments, and personal possessions to the exclusion of social and spiritual characteristics, as indicated by at least five of the following:

a. beliefs that things are the most important reality in the world

b. acts as if physical wellbeing is the highest value in the world

c. considers the physical world as people's main concern

d. explains everything as it concerns money

e. rejects intellectual, social or spiritual values

f. centers her thinking on money and investments

g. assumes that life is the result of a natural process

h. finds excessive satisfaction in shopping.

The materialistic disorder is in complete contrast to spiritual living. While the material focuses on the physical, the spiritual focuses on the things of the spirit.

2.32 Characteristics of Materialistic Disorder

Associated Features and Coexisting Disorders

This disorder is commonly related to the self-centered disorder, since materialists often see their possessions and money as an extension of themselves. They are what they have.

Onset Age and History

Materialism develops early in children as they accumulate excessive amounts of toys and things. As people grow up, many learn that the effort to keep up their toys is greater than the benefit they derive from them. Nevertheless, materialism is common and a great barrier to spiritual growth.

Impairment in Social and Occupational Functions

People with this disorder limit their social relationships and hinder the occupations. Material things take an excessive important place in their lives. The materials are their higher power.

Prevalence Range

Persons without an active spiritual life tend to be materialistic. Their lives focus on the things they can see. They claim that the unseen is not real to them.

2.33 Materialistic Martha

Martha values the things she can see and hold and ignores most everything else. Material things give her certainty, and help her deal with her needs. She cannot count, hold, sell, buy, or accumulate spiritual issues, but material things she can. To her, they seem more real.

Martha has developed a great love of money, investments, books, and jewelry. Since she has quite an accumulation of them, they give her a feeling of superiority and security. She does not realize that she may lose all of them, and may have to start all over again. What comes, goes.

Her problem with materialism is the fact that it crowds out so many other areas of life. She is selfish. She would enjoy art, music, writing, and friendship much more if she would not evaluate everything in the context of money.

Where would you start helping Martha?

___ Encourage her to give some of her possessions away to people who really need them to live.

___ Make an inventory of her non-material possessions.

___ Consider adding to her life a spiritual dimension.

Moshe Dyan, Israel's General, is reported to have said, "They don't make statues for people who make a lot of money, but for those who give it away."

2.34 People Will Love only their Money

Lexis De Tocqueville, the noted French historian, wrote in the 1840s: "The love of wealth is...at the bottom of all that the Americans do." This world is indeed very materialistic. The love of money is the mast common materialist love. While there are other forms of materialism, the value of most physical material is finally expressed in the form of money.

There are some, who value money more than relationships. Many families are torn apart at the death of a father over the money that he has left behind for his family. The money seems more important than the family.

There are people who will do anything for money. Their love of money is greater than any other love or value. They cannot understand any other wealth beside material riches. However, money is not the most valuable item in the universe. People acquire and lose it, and life goes on. Overall, people with plenty of money usually are not happier than people with little money.

The possession of money gives a false sense of security. Issues of relationships, health, and peace of mind are far more important than financial security. We are secure when we have peace of mind and caring relationships. It is true that money frees one to pursue various interests. In that, it is a means to an end, not an end in itself. We have a materialist disorder, when we place the value our possessions above the value of our relationships with God and others.

2.35 Secular

The secular pertains to worldly things, or to things that are not regarded as religious, spiritual, sacred, or eternal. The majority of people is secular and makes no or little room for spiritual living.

Thus, in a way, the secular is the opposite of the spiritual. The material around us is very worldly. This part of our world is only temporary.

There is a place for both the materialistic and the secular. We live in a material world that is built out of the physical. Nobody can deny that. Nevertheless, just because our world is physical, does not exclude the spiritual. There is no dichotomy, there is room for the physical and the spiritual.

Secular people can have spiritual disorders. Some of these disorders concern themselves with life priorities, purpose, and values that are philosophical and secular.

Materialism as such is nearly always secular. It denies the importance of things beyond the material. Communism is one of the expressions of materialism. Communists concern themselves primarily with the distribution of material things and deny the existence of spiritual life.

Perhaps the term secular comes from the concept that the spiritual is primary and the material secondary. Its root meaning is "temporal." We come into this world with a soul, but no external physical possessions.

2.36 Hodge, S. R. (1949, October). **Men, Machines, and Materialism,** *Br Med J.*

"Inevitably there arise in the tides of men's affairs issues which demand attention. Wars and their accompanying problems call for direct action, and commonly the men and the means are found and the resources of the people are urgently deployed. There follows almost inevitably a period of relative exhaustion and uncertainty... With the threat of physical extinction or subjection, we have grappled not once but again, and with a remarkable unanimity and singleness of purpose. To minimize the eroding effect on a civilization of two major wars in one generation would be futile, but the contemplation of certain human trends -trends which display the 'inevitability of gradualness' and a malignant persistence-cannot fail to be gravely disturbing."

"Not the least of our perils lies in our own approach to this spreading cult of materialism. Scientific method induces us to weigh and to analyze evidence and motive, and there is a compelling charm in these procedures, which may blind us to the fact of our essential humanity and to the existence of the incommunicable, which go to make it. Study of the computing machine and allied mechanisms may help us to greater understanding of those cerebral mechanisms which are explainable in such terms, and 'analysis' (in the psycho-analytic sense) has afforded and may continue to afford us greater insight into the motivation of human behavior. But the ' analytic situation' and the 'mechanistic analogy' may assume disproportionate significance, and paralysis of action with spiritual sterility ensues."

2.37 Whybrow, Peter. (2005). **American Mania: When More Is Not Enough.** *MedGenMed.* 7(3): 70. Reviewed by Hayes Virginia M. and Zylowska Lidia.

"Peter Whybrow's, MD, groundbreaking book, *American Mania: When More Is Not Enough*, is the first work to approach the American national obsession with materialism and overconsumption from the multiple perspectives of economics, philosophy, psychology, and neurobiology."

"The author makes an analogy between the frantic pursuit of material goods and the cyclic phases of bipolar disorder observed in patients. Dr. Whybrow compares the economic boom of the 1990s to the happy, elated, and overly optimistic mood of an early manic phase; the resulting economic irresponsibility and overspending are paralleled to the irritable manic phase that finally ends with the inevitable reckoning of the depressive phase."

"Integrating findings from interviews and observations, *American Mania* depicts us as a nation living in a frantic pursuit of more: a bigger house, a faster car, and the latest in 'new, improved' merchandise. Chronically overworked and on the go, Americans are driving themselves to exhaustion, spending less quality time with themselves, their friends, and their families. Dr. Whybrow warns that there is a physical and psychological price to pay: Rates of anxiety, depression, and self-destructive behaviors, including obesity and addiction, are higher today than ever and appear to increase with each new generation."

2.4 Pleasure-seeking Disorder

SD4

2.41 Spiritual Pleasure-seeking Disorder

A lifestyle centered on the personal pursuit of pleasure (hedonism), and the avoidance of pain as the main good in life, as indicated by at least three of the following:

a. avoids all that interferes with his personal pleasure

b. reduces his pain at all costs

c. pursues a life of pleasure

d. spends most of his resources on pleasure

e. looks for pleasure in all aspects of living

f. considers food, sports and entertainment as life's main concerns

g. Seeks constantly pleasures related to sex or sports.

To the pleasure-seeker, pleasure becomes the focus and god that controls everything. A true pleasure-seeker has no spiritual life. Pleasure-seeking in all its forms may become an addiction.

Whereas SD1, joylessness, is a deficit of pleasure, pleasure-seeking is an excess of pleasure.

2.42 Characteristics of Pleasure-seeking Disorder

Associated Features and Coexisting Disorders

For many, continuous pleasure-seeking is the higher power that organizes their lives. Thus, other spiritual disorders follow in their wake. For many, the materialistic is their highest pleasure. Addiction is often a coexisting disorder.

Besides being a spiritual disorder, pleasure-seeking has psychological, social, and physical components. It affects all parts of life. It makes living in a healthy spiritual climate impossible. It limits life to such an extent that spirituality cannot blossom.

Some people are controlled not by their values or objectives, but by their disorders and addictions. They give up the most important part of their lives, their priorities, and life objectives.

Associated Features and Coexisting Disorders

Pleasure-seeking may grow into a spiritual disorder that is related to the mental disorder of addiction. In some cases, both disorders may require treatment.

Onset Age and History

Like the self-centered disorder, pleasure-seeking starts at infancy and either takes its reasonable place in childhood and adulthood, or it keeps growing and dominates life. For most, pleasure-seeking peaks at ages 20-45 and then starts to decline.

Impairment in Social and occupations functions

Pleasure-seeking is very self-centered and thus inhibits social relationships. Most people work for money, rather than the joy of working. They find little or no pleasure in work.

Prevalence Range

Pleasure seeking is prevalent among those with a higher standard of living, who do not have to worry where they will find their next meal. They will invest all their resources in their pleasure-seeking disorder. On the other hand, the flower children, who have nothing, may also use all they find in pleasure-seeking.

2.43 Pleasurable Peter

Early in life, Peter had to make some big choices. Would he focus his life on becoming rich, famous, or helpful, or on just having fun? He was not a materialist and money held little interest for him. He did not care if people thought him to be great and outstanding. He did not see himself as a doctor who would help people get well. However, the last one was a consideration.

Peter chose to have fun. Most of it was good clean fun. He saw nothing wrong in following the sports, and he was an enthusiastic fan of his teams. When possible, he attended the games and wore the team colors. He enjoyed many sports and his team-mates were his best friends.

Peter avoided everything that brought no immediate pleasure. He could advance in some aspects of life, but many were just too hard work to pursue. They just were not fun.

How could you help broaden Peter's life?

__ Help him inventory the fun and non-fun parts of his life.

__ Help him explore some areas of life that he had considered as no fun that by now may be fun.

__ Help him learn to put up with some pain.

2.44 The Good and Bad of Pleasure

Most of us enjoy life and find pleasure in our families, our friends, our eating. Life has its pleasures and we appreciate them.

In some areas of life, the lack of pleasure can be very frustrating. Some people find no pleasure in their life partners, their religion, their work and their health. Their lack of pleasure in specific instances can move them away from what they have and seek what they lack. Sometimes they find it; often it is just a change of venues that does little to bring pleasure.

Sometimes that seeking after pleasure becomes a life priority. Some discard anything that is not pleasurable. Nevertheless, some things in life are not pleasurable; they have to be done to live.

When pleasure-seeking becomes a priority, it also manifests itself as a spiritual disorder. Service is not always pleasurable, but if we stop serving others, we fold in on ourselves and lose all the pleasure of life. When we become self-centered or selfish, we miss so many opportunities to relate to others and service-connected pleasures.

Pleasure can be good or bad dependent on its place in our lives. It is a pleasure to serve God and man. But if we do it only for our pleasure, we miss the pleasure.

2.45 Joy and Pleasure

There is a close relationship between the first spiritual disorder (SD1) and the fourth one (SD4). We cannot be spiritually healthy without the normal joy of living. That joy helps us cope with many difficult situations and depressions.

A person who finds no pleasure in living is in real difficulty. Life can lose its meaning and purpose. Life can become so dark that no joyous light can penetrate it.

Therefore finding your joy in life is important and necessary to healthy living. However, it is unhealthy to focus your life on specific pleasures to the exclusion of others.

We may derive pleasure from serving others. Not being able to find pleasure in service may be a spiritual joylessness disorder (SD1). But seeking pleasure mainly in service to clients may be a spiritual pleasure-seeking disorder (SD4), if it dominates life and is associated with other spiritual disorders.

It comes down to the place of joy and pleasure in life. They are both needed, but can cause problems if they are too rare or too dominant. All spiritual disorders are found on a continuum. We need a limited amount of self-concern, but self-centeredness is a disorder. We need a limited amount of material concerns, but materialism is a spiritual disorder.

2.46 Berridge, Kent, C., and Kringelbach, Morten L. (2011, October 12). **Building a neuroscience of pleasure and well-being.** *Psychol Well Being.* 1(1): 1–3.

"First, what is pleasure? Pleasure is never merely a sensation, even for sensory pleasures. Instead, it always requires the recruitment of specialized pleasure-generating brain systems to paint an additional 'hedonic gloss' onto a sensation. Active recruitment of brain pleasure-generating systems is what makes a pleasant experience 'liked'".

"The capacity of certain stimuli, such as a sweet taste or a loved one, to reliably elicit pleasure – to nearly always be painted with a hedonic gloss – reflects the privileged ability of such stimuli to activate those hedonic brain systems responsible for manufacturing and applying the gloss. Hedonic brain systems are well-developed in the brain, spanning subcortical and cortical levels, and are quite similar across humans and other animals."

"Some might be surprised by high similarity across species, or by substantial subcortical contributions, at least if one thinks of pleasure as uniquely human and as emerging only at the top of the brain. Pleasure as an adaptive feature is not so hard to imagine. For example, tasty food is one of the most universal routes to pleasure, as well as an essential requirement to survival."

"Beyond food, sex is another potent and adaptive sensory pleasure which involves some of the same brain circuits."

2.5 Fear Disorder

SD5

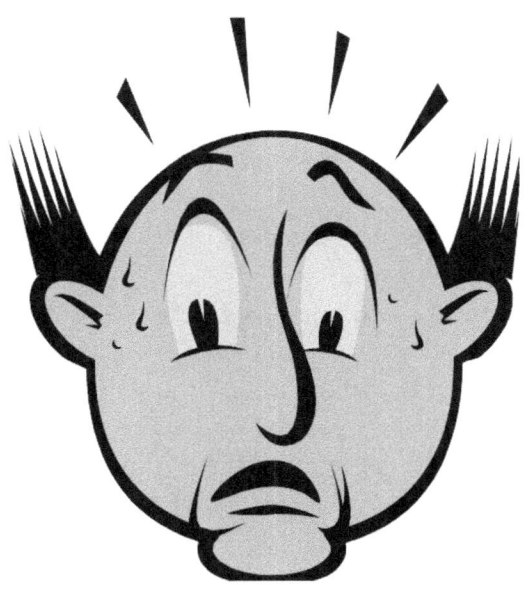

2.51 Spiritual Fear Disorder

Fear alerts a person of possible danger to come. In that, it is normal and useful. It also prepares a person for a situation that requires high respect or complex relationships. However, when the alarm bells go off often in a day without a good reason, there is a disorder somewhere. One of the common spiritual fears is the fear of death. Many people do not have a clear answer to the question, 'What happens when we die?' Fear disorder is indicated by at least four of the following:

a. reacts continually with fear when there is no basis for fear

b. approaches everything new or unknown with fear

c. accepts the loss of relationships or possessions fearfully

d. expresses her fears through anger

e. expresses strongly her fear of death

f. talks often about her fear of loss

g. deals much with situations that express worry and anxiety.

In fear, we believe that something bad will happen and that we are defenseless against it. We worry. In fear, we experience the evil before it actually happens. In a way, in fear we walk through the anticipated harm, in joy we walk through the coming good.

2.52 Characteristics of Fear Disorder

Associated Features and Coexisting Disorders

Some people feel falsely that they have done something wrong when in actuality the wrong was not their fault. There are sometimes good reasons for a person to feel guilty, but at other times, that feeling is not warranted.

Onset Age and History

Children often develop unjustified fears that stay with them, sometimes for a long time, sometimes throughout life. Some fears develop in the later parts of life. Most people outlive their childhood fears and go on to a normal life.

Impairment in Social and occupations functions

Fear can paralyze persons and thus hinder their relationships. Fear in one area can carry over to other areas, including the fear of intimate relationships.

Prevalence Range

The fear disorder is quite common in individuals who have a vivid imagination. They can find fears where there is nothing to fear.

2.53 Fearful Fern

Fern has so much going for her. She is part of a loving family, has good friends, and is very satisfied with her work. Her income is adequate, and nobody is suing her.

However, Fern is not at peace. She is haunted by fears that she can hardly describe. She worries about many things. She is anxious. She asks herself constantly the question: "What would I do if..."

Of course, the "if" never happens. Life goes on rather well. Her fears cast a negative cloud over all her life. She cannot enjoy what are obvious blessings. There seem to be no reasons that would support her fears.

Fern's fears seem to be the product of a restless mind. In addition, she likes perfection and nothing seems to be perfect. The pictures of disaster are so real in her mind and the portraits of peace so far.

Where would you start helping Fern?

___ Point out the unreasonableness of her fears.

___ Help her find real and imaginary places of peace.

___ Help her make peace with God by requesting forgiveness.

2.54 Fear of Old Age and Death

King Solomon wrote a pessimistic description of old age in Ecclesiastes 12:1-7. However, people can face it with courage.

"1 ***Remember now your Creator*** in the days of your youth, while the evil days (of old age) come not, nor the years draw nigh, when thou shall say, I have no pleasure in them;   2 While the sun, or the light, or the moon, or the stars, be not darkened (while you can see), nor the clouds return after the rain (always dark): 3 In the day when the keepers of the house (hands and feet) shall tremble, and the strong men shall bow themselves (stooped), and the grinders (teeth) cease because they are few, and those that look out of the windows be darkened (can't see), 4 And the doors shall be shut in the streets (sick and alone), when the sound of the grinding is low (can't hear), and he shall rise up at the voice of the bird (awake easily), and all the daughters of music shall be brought low (can's hear); 5 Also when they shall be afraid of that which is high (no use of ladders), and fears shall be in the way, and the almond tree (white hair) shall flourish, and the grasshopper shall be a burden (no strength), and desire shall fail (no taste and sex): because man goes to his long home (death), and the mourners go about the streets: 6 Or ever the silver cord (marrow of back bone) be loosed, or the golden bowl (membrane of brain) be broken, or the pitcher (heart chambers) be broken at the fountain, or the wheel (arteries) broken at the cistern. 7 Then shall the dust return to the earth as it was and the spirit shall return unto God who gave it. 8 Vanity of vanities, said the preacher; all is vanity."

2.55 Cicirelli, Victor G., Gerontol J. (2009, January). **Sibling Death and Death Fear in Relation to Depressive Symptomatology in Older Adults.** Sci *Soc Sci*. 64B(1): 24–32

"Previously overlooked factors in elders' depressive symptomatology were examined, including death fear, sibling death, and sibling closeness. Participants were 150 elders (61 men, 89 women) aged 65–97 years with at least one sibling. Measures were proportion of deceased siblings, sibling closeness, the Death Fear Subscale of the Death Attitude Profile–Revised, and the Center for Epidemiological Studies–Depression scale (20-item adult form). Death fear, sibling closeness, and proportion of dead siblings were directly related to depression, with path coefficients of .42, −.24, and .13, respectively. Proportion of dead siblings had indirect effects on depression, as did age and education. Depressive symptomatology in old age is influenced by death fear related to sibling death as well as by poor relationships with them; it must be understood within a situational context including death fear and sibling relationships."

"Death fear can be defined as an emotional reaction to perceptions of one's own inevitable mortality, involving feelings of helplessness in the face of this threat to one's existence. In general, fear of death gradually declines from young adulthood to late middle age, remaining relatively low but stable throughout old age, despite the fact that many elders appear to develop an acceptance of death. Yet, considerable individual differences in elders' fear of death exist, with many reporting substantial fear."

2.56 Boscarino, Joseph, Adams, E Richard, Figley Charles R., Galea, Sanro, and Foa Edna B. (2009 June 23). **Fear of Terrorism and Preparedness in New York City 2 Years After the Attacks: Implications for Disaster Planning and Research.** *J Public Health Manag Pract. PMC*

"We conducted a random cross-sectional survey of 1,681 adults interviewed 2 years after the WTCD. Participants were living in New York City at the time of the attack and exposed to ongoing terrorist threats."

"We found 44.9 percent (95% confidence interval [CI] = 41.9–47.9) of residents were concerned about future attacks and 16.9 percent (95% CI = 14.7–19.3) reported a fear level of '10' on a 10-point analog scale. Furthermore, 14.8 percent (95% CI = 12.8–17.0) reported they had made some plans for a future attack, a significant increase from the previous year."

"In addition, although 42.6 percent (95% CI = 39.6–45.7) indicated that they would likely wait for evacuation instructions following a chemical, biological, or nuclear attack, 34.4 percent (95% CI = 31.5–37.3) reported they would evacuate immediately against official advice."

"Our study suggests that among those exposed to ongoing terrorism threats, terrorism fear, and preparedness were related to socioeconomic factors, mental health status, terrorism exposure levels, and exposure to stressful life events."

"Research in both animal models and humans has enabled the development of an initial model of the neurocircuitry supporting the regulation of conditioned fear. There is a network of brain regions hypothesized to support fear regulation through the four methods discussed in this review—extinction, cognitive regulation, active coping, and reconsolidation. Despite the fact that cognitive techniques may be deployed intentionally, unlike the relatively passive learning that takes place during extinction, the neural substrates supporting cognitive regulation appear to overlap in part with the regions involved in diminishing fear through extinction. Both extinction and cognitive regulation seem to use prefrontal inhibitory mechanisms to regulate amygdale-driven fear expression."

"Active coping and reconsolidation are two methods of fear regulation that are presently less well understood. Taking instrumental action to reduce exposure to fear-inducing contexts and stimuli is something we do regularly in our everyday lives. Active coping seems to be an important means of controlling fear that has not yet been widely incorporated in clinical practice. Reconsolidation is an especially promising method of regulating fear, as its effects seem to be more robust, in that fear responses are less likely to reemerge. Active coping and reconsolidation may provide avenues for regulating fear under conditions in which these methods are rendered ineffective."

Even when things look bad and we have reasons to fear, we can have peace of mind and face the future with confidence.

2.6 Unforgiveness Disorder

SD6

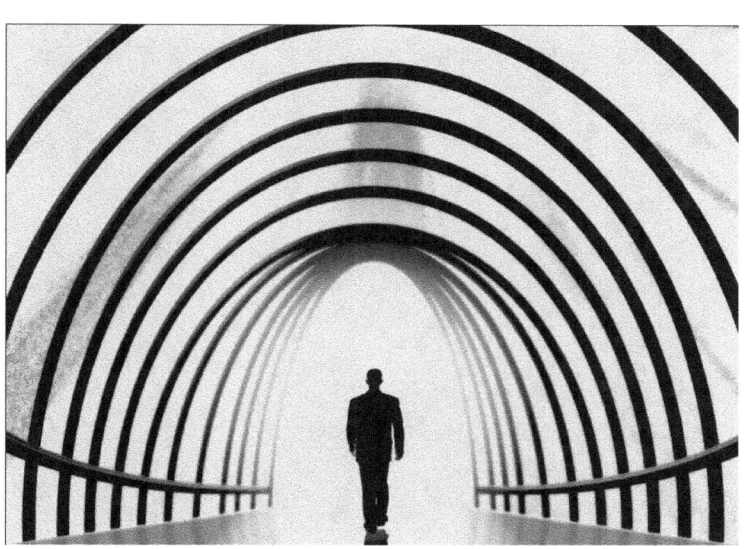

2.61 Spiritual Unforgiveness Disorder

Forgiveness is central to the spiritual life. Without it, we experience many of the other spiritual disorders. Without it, we lose our joy, our altruism and love, our ability to give and serve our peace. Unforgiveness disorder is indicated by at least three of the following:

a. refrains from forgiving others for their mistakes

b. retains grudges and desires for revenge

 c. refuses to accept forgiveness from others

d. refuses to forgive himself

e. feels no need to forgive

f. feels no need to be forgiven.

Forgiveness is a powerful healer of bad situations. Unforgiveness on the other hand reinforces the bad situation.

The Bible asks us to forgive: "Forgive one another, even as God for Christ's sake has forgiven you." Ephesians 4:32

2.62 Characteristics of Unforgiveness Disorder

Associated Features and Coexisting Disorders

Unforgiveness is a form of self-centeredness, where anything that would possibly weaken self is perceived as a threat. A self-centered person is not able to forgive, because he or she feels that they must get even with any offender. In addition, a materialistic person values the materialistic so highly that they cannot give up any of it.

Onset Age and History

Children generally forgive easily. It is when they become teens and adults, and when relationships become more complex, that forgiveness becomes harder. At one time, some divorced people might not have been able to forgive and thus broke their marriage.

Prevalence Range

The great majority of people have some individuals whom they have not fully forgiven. That may not rise to the level of a mild disorder, but it may affect relationships. People who pray usually ask God for forgiveness of their sins and mistakes,

2.63 Unforgiving Frank

Frank is controlled by the people he cannot forgive. There is his ex-wife, his former boss, his children who are estranged. He feels that the world is not fair. Moreover, he set out to take revenge on all who hurt him.

It does not seem to work. Frank feels more hurt than the people he tries to get even with and hurt. His attacks on them seem to roll off from them, but they stick to him. He feels very alone. The people who used to be close to him are now afraid of him and keep their distance.

Frank does not understand when people talk about a forgiving God. To Frank, God is the judge that destroys the ones that do wrong. How does forgiveness fit into that?

Where would you start as you help Frank to forgive?

__ Point out that much of the hurt is his fault.

__ Explain how Christ died to forgive Frank's sins.

__ Help him to reconnect with his ex-wife.

2.64 Unforgivable Sin

Some people think that their lack of forgiveness and spirituality is because they have committed the unpardonable sin mentioned by Christ in Matthew 12: 30-33 and Mark 3:20-30.

"Matthew 12:30. He that is not with me is against me; and he that gathers not with me scatters abroad. 31 Wherefore I say unto you, all manner of sin and blasphemy shall be forgiven unto men: but the blasphemy against the Holy Ghost shall not be forgiven unto men.

32 And whosoever speaks a word against the Son of man, it shall be forgiven him: but whosoever speaks against the Holy Ghost, it shall not be forgiven him, neither in this world, neither in the world to come. 33 Either make the tree good, and his fruit good; or else make the tree corrupt, and his fruit corrupt: for the tree is known by his fruit."

Many believe that the unpardonable sin (the blasphemy against the Holy Spirit) is the habitual calling of something good evil, and the evil good. People who are concerned about whether they have committed the unpardonable sin have not committed it. Their concern may show that they are in a relationship with God who forgives sin. It may be that some of those who do not deal with this issue call the loving Lord a harsh and unloving judge.

2.65 The Forgiven

In the Lord's Prayer, people pray to God for forgiveness from their sins. To them, forgiveness is a requirement for a healthy relationship with God. Unforgiveness creates a barrier between them and God. Only God can remove that barrier. God grants forgiveness to all who trust him and follow him. Not all the good that good people do removes that barrier.

Central to God's forgiveness of our evil is our willingness to forgive the evil of others. Forgiveness becomes an attitude that connects us to others and to God.

Forgiveness resolves guilt and promotes healing. Conflicts, negatives, depression, self-centeredness, materialism, and fear all disappear when love flows freely between individuals and God. The healing oil lubricates all interactions.

Forgiveness is a free gift from God, that comes to us without conditions. We cannot earn it. We can only appreciate it, and accept it. It is the soil, in which a strong spiritual life grows.

All spiritual disorders separate people from their God. The joy-less lack a bridge to God. So do the selfish, materialistic, fearful, unforgiving, and dishonesty. Christians see Christ as that bridge. Forgiveness provides that connection. The healing of spiritual disorders does not only free people to live fully here and now, but also to enjoy God's creation without limitations of time and space.

2.66 Harris, Alex H. S. and Thorsen, Carl E. (2005) **Forgiveness, Unforgiveness, Health, and Disease, Retrieved from** http://www.chce.research.va.gov/docs/pdfs/pi_publications/Harris/2005_Harris_Thorsen_HF.pdf

"Five years ago, we observed that no evidence existed from controlled studies linking forgiveness to physiology, health, or disease. Since then, the theory, measurement, and empirical study of forgiveness have developed substantially. Evidence has been produced, linking both forgiveness and unforgiveness to short-term physiological variables, such as cortical reactivity, blood pressure, and skin conductance. Coupled with the related literature on stress and health, this evidence makes hypotheses directly linking unforgiveness and forgiveness with health and disease variables more plausible, and ripe to be tested. However, direct evidence that forgiveness or unforgiveness are related to health or disease is still virtually nonexistent. We review hypotheses and theoretical models linking forgiveness and unforgiveness to health and disease, and we present supporting evidence where available."

"Unforgiveness has been defined by Worthington and colleagues) as a combination of delayed negative emotions (i.e., resentment, bitterness, hostility, hatred, anger, and fear) toward a transgressor. We view unforgiveness essentially as stress response with potential health consequences."

"Not everyone who experiences an offense experiences unforgiveness. Forgiveness can be seen as one of many ways to reduce or avoid unforgiveness. As such, the hypothesized health benefits of reducing unforgiveness and fostering forgiveness are not necessarily synonymous. We view forgiveness not only as the reduction of unforgiveness through reducing the negative thoughts, emotions, motivations, and behaviors toward the offender, but also as the increase of positive emotions and perspectives, such as empathy, hope, or compassion.'

"We consider three general hypotheses that are relevant to the notion that forgiveness and unforgiveness may be related to physical health and disease; (a) Unforgiveness is associated with health risks; (b) positive states that are characteristic of forgiveness have health benefits beyond those associated with the reduction of unforgiveness; and (c) forgiveness interventions produce changes in health and disease outcomes when evaluated with randomized trials."

The story goes that the famous Russian psychologist Pavel Pailov Pavlotski was able to teach people to forgive the most hideous crimes by just drawing daily pictures of the compassion expressed by the forgiver. The story of course is fiction. There never was a Pavel Pailov Pavlotski nor a picture therapy like this. Forgiveness takes more than that.

Forgiveness requires spiritual awareness, spiritual receptivity, and spiritual response. Some lessons on how to acquire these are found in Part Three of this volume.

2.7 Dishonesty Disorder

SD7

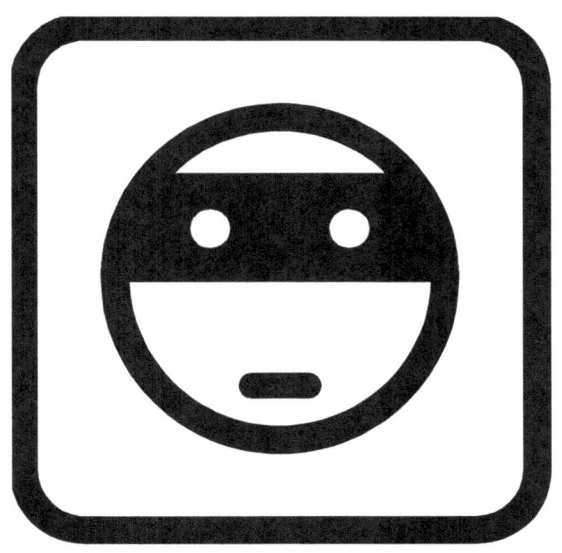

2.71 Spiritual Dishonesty Disorder

Dishonest behaviors include violation of social and spiritual laws and crimes like homicide, assault, rape, robbery, theft, embezzlement, and burglary. It is the habitual falsehood, doing wrong, and lack of integrity, such as lying, cheating, deceiving, and stealing, as indicated by at least three of the following:

a. lacks the ability to communicate truth

b. manifests corrupt thinking or behavior

c. avoids or misrepresents reality

d. deceives others with or without a specific purpose

e. steals habitually

f. cheats habitually.

Honesty is based on reality, dishonesty on fantasy. In dishonesty, the offenders things that they can fool the hearer into believing their made-up story.

2.72 Characteristics of Dishonesty Disorder

Associated Features and Coexisting Disorders

Dishonesty behavior is often associated with the self-centeredness disorders, for they come from the same root. Both ignore the order that comes from submission to a higher power or to laws designed to keep relationships in order.

Onset Age and History

Some children develop this disorder early and give it up in their teens. There are some individuals who get addicted to dishonesty, and who make criminal behavior their lifestyle.

Impairment in Social and occupations functions

Dishonesty limits all social relationships because a dishonest person cannot be trusted. Without trust, relationships die.

Prevalence Range

In some societies, dishonesty runs deep; in others, it is rather rare.

2.73 Dishonest Dick

It has not been easy for Dick to survive in his neighborhood. There were drugs, shooting and gangs. Just to come and go from his parent's home each day was dangerous and difficult.

Dick did not know any honest people. It seemed that all people around him stole, lied, and cheated. He could not even trust his parents and siblings.

The evil world was pressing heavily onto Dick. Dishonesty seemed to be his only defense in that world. He often could not remember his previous lies and thus messed things up worse. There was nobody to help him.

Most middle-aged men he knew had served time in prison. There they had learned more ways that are deceptive. In that, they were experts. Dave had no idea of truth.

Where would you start helping Dave?

__ Help him understand the evil of deceit.

__ Help him differentiate between good and evil.

__ Teach him to love somebody in order to be honest with him or her.

2.74 Dishonesty and Choice

People make a clear choice to be either honest or dishonest. Honesty is related to reality and to what is actually happening. Dishonesty is connected with deception and a desire to portray a willful picture, a dream, or a fantasy. Dishonesty may sound good, but the things dishonesty talks about are not actually there.

Much of dishonesty is partial dishonesty. There is often enough truth in the description to gain the confidence of the listener, and enough lie in the description to hurt her. Truth and dishonesty do not mix. Dishonesty mixed with truth is still dishonesty.

People talk about gray areas as if there were half-truths and half-lies. In reality, nothing here is half-and-half. Anything touched by dishonesty is dishonest.

Today most populations are so used to deception that they do not recognize it as the evil that it really is. Their thinking-home is deception. Without thinking, they depart from reality and enlarge on the truth in order to appear greater than they are.

Yet there are many who have as their thinking home the truth. They realize the evil of deception and avoid it all costs. Their conscience is educated to guide their choices.

2.75 Sip, Kamila E., Skewes, Joshua C., Marchant, Jennifer. L., McGregor, William B., Roepstorff, Andreas, and Frith, Christopher D. (2012) **What if I Get Busted? Deception, Choice, and Decision-Making in Social Interaction**. *Front Neurosci*. 6: 58.

"Deception is an essentially social act, yet little is known about how social consequences affect the decision to deceive. In this study, participants played a computerized game of deception without constraints on whether or when to attempt to deceive their opponent. Participants were questioned by an opponent outside the scanner about their knowledge of the content of a display. Importantly, questions were posed so that, in some conditions, it was possible to be deceptive, while in other conditions it was not. To simulate a realistic interaction, participants could be confronted about their claims by the opponent. This design, therefore, creates a context in which a deceptive participant runs the risk of being punished if their deception is detected."

"Our results show that participants were slower to give honest than to give deceptive responses when they knew more about the display, and could use this knowledge for their own benefit. The condition in which confrontation was not possible was associated with increased activity in subgeneral anterior cingulated cortex. The processing of a question that allows a deceptive response was associated with activation in right caudate and inferior frontal gyros. Our findings suggest the decision to deceive is affected by the potential risk of social confrontation rather than the claim itself."

2.76 Mead, Nicole L., Baumeister F., Gino, Francesca, Schweitzer,Maurixe E., and Ariely Dan. (2009). **Too Tired to Tell the Truth: Self-Control Resource Depletion and Dishonesty.** *J Exp Soc Psychol.* 45(3): 594–597.

"The opportunity to profit from dishonesty evokes a motivational conflict between the temptation to cheat for selfish gain, and the desire to act in a socially appropriate manner. Honesty may depend on self-control, given that self-control is the capacity that enables people to override antisocial selfish responses in favor of socially desirable responses. Two experiments tested the hypothesis that dishonesty would increase when people's self-control resources were depleted by an initial act of self-control. Depleted participants misrepresented their performance for monetary gain to a greater extent than did non-depleted participants (Experiment 1). Perhaps more troubling, depleted participants were more likely than non-depleted participants to expose themselves to the temptation to cheat, thereby aggravating the effects of depletion on cheating (Experiment 2). Results indicate that dishonesty increases when people's capacity to exert self-control is impaired."

"When given the opportunity to profit from a dishonest act, what determines whether people cheat or remain honest? Such opportunities present a motivational conflict between taking short-term, selfish gain, and acting in virtuous ways that presumably bring long-term rewards that include social acceptance. Resolving such dilemmas may be one of the core functions of self-control."

2.77 Talwar, Victoria, Gordon, Lee, Heidi, Kang M. (2007, May) **Lying in the Elementary School Years.** *Dev Psychol.* 43(3): 804–810.

"The development of lying to conceal one's own transgression was examined in school-age children. Children (N = 172) between 6 and 11 years of age were asked not to peek at the answer to a trivia question while left alone in a room. Half of the children could not resist temptation and peeked at the answer. When the experimenter asked them whether they had peeked, the majority of children lied. However, children's subsequent verbal statements, made in response to follow-up questioning, were not always consistent with their initial denial and, hence, leaked critical information to reveal their deceit. Children's ability to maintain consistency between their initial lie and subsequent verbal statements increased with age."

"Lying, in essence, is theory of mind in action. Lying refers to the act by which one deliberately makes a false statement with intent to instill false beliefs into the mind of the statement's recipient. To lie successfully, lie-tellers must be able to have an appropriate assessment of their own and the recipients' mental states. Lie-tellers must then construct and produce false statements that differ from their true beliefs about the state of affairs. Further, the false statements must be carefully constructed such that they will not arouse suspicion in the recipient. This often requires lie-tellers to produce verbal and nonverbal behaviors that are consistent with the false statement but inconsistent with their true beliefs and to conceal beliefs incongruent with the false statement."

2.8 Unspecified Disorder

SD8

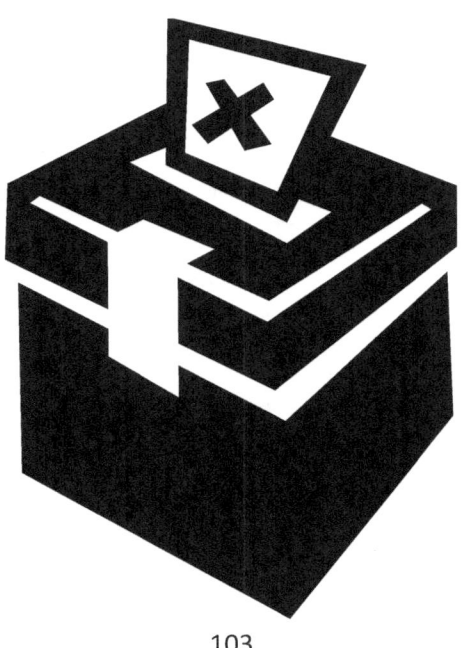

2.81 Spiritual Unspecified Disorder

A healthy person has a balanced active physical, mental, social, and spiritual life. When one of these areas does not perform well, he or she is ill. One of the common spiritual disorders is the minimizing of one of these areas, particularly the spiritual one. Spiritual disorders may include various addictions, judgementalism, intemperance, and different manifestations of unkindness and unthankfulness. A person with the spiritual unspecified disorder has four of the traits below:

a. denies the existence of a God or a spiritual world

b. makes spiritual life a very low priority

c. criticizes spiritual people as unrealistic

d. is unable to find satisfaction in spiritual living

e. refuses to activate her spiritual insights

f. lives with addiction or intemperance

g. lives with habitual unkindness.

"The Order of the Divine mind, embodied in the Divine Law, is beautiful. What should a man do but try to reproduce it, as far as possible, in his daily life?" C. S. Lewis, *Reflections on the Psalms,* p. 59.

2.82 Verghese, Abraham. (2008, October-December). **Spirituality and mental health.** *Indian J Psychiatry.* 50(4): 233–237.

"Spirituality is a globally acknowledged concept. It involves belief and obedience to an all-powerful force usually called God, who controls the universe and the destiny of man. It involves the ways in which people fulfill what they hold to be the purpose of their lives, a search for the meaning of life and a sense of connectedness to the universe. The universality of spirituality extends across creed and culture. At the same time, spirituality is very much personal and unique to each person. It is a sacred realm of human experience. Spirituality produces in man qualities such as love, honesty, patience, tolerance, compassion, a sense of detachment, faith, and hope."

"Religion is institutionalized spirituality. Thus, there are several religions having different sets of beliefs, traditions, and doctrines. They have different types of community-based worship programs. Spirituality is the common factor in all these religions. It is possible that religions can lose their spirituality when they become institutions of oppression instead of agents of goodwill, peace, and harmony. They can become divisive instead of unifying. History will tell us that this had happened from time to time. It has been said that more blood has been shed in the cause of religion than any other cause. The medieval holy wars of Europe, the religion-based terrorism and conflicts of modern times are examples. We must remember that the institutions of religion are supposed to help us to practice spirituality in our lives."

2.83 Smith, David B. (2007, May 15) **Addiction as a Spiritual Disease,** *Articlesbase,* <www.articlesbase.com/religion-articles/addiction-as-a-spiritual-disease-147644.html.>

"Addiction is a spiritual disease. Because addiction is a direct assault against the Self, it is also a direct attack on the spirit or soul of the person suffering from the addiction. A person's spirit sustains life; addiction leads to spiritual death."

"One of most tragic consequences of an addictive condition is the way it can destroy the heart and soul of a beautiful person. Whether the problem is drugs, alcohol, sex, gambling, or work, the common pattern is that as the addictive personality gains more and more control of the addict, the person loses more and more of their ability to influence their own thoughts and behavior. In the process, a spiritual deadening takes place."

"Here the definition of 'spiritual' involves being connected in a meaningful way to the world. It involves having the ability to extract meaning from one's experiences. The feeling of belonging and being an important part of the world is lost as addiction progresses. The sense of knowing oneself and one's value drifts farther and farther away."

"Addiction is a spiritual disease. Everybody has the ability to connect with the soul and spirit of others, and it is indeed these deeper relationships that the addict desperately needs. However, because addiction is a direct assault against the Self, it is also a direct attack on the spirit or soul of the person suffering from the addiction. A person's spirit sustains life; addiction leads to spiritual death."

"The longer the addiction goes on, the more spiritually isolated the person becomes. This is the saddest and most frightening aspect of addiction. Sunsets, smiles, laughter, support from others, and other things that nourish the spirit come to mean less as acting out becomes more important."

"Because addiction blocks a person's ability to effectively connect with his or her own spirit, there is little chance to connect with the spirit of others. Relationships with others become more superficial as the illness progresses. Addicts stay isolated or turn to the presence of other addicts who offer companionship and little or no fear of confrontation."

"As addiction progresses, spiritual deadening deepens. This may be the most dangerous aspect of addiction. For recovery to begin there must be a recommitment to the nurturing of one's spirit. The farther one moves away from the Self, the harder it is to reestablish a healing relationship."

"In the beginning of the addictive process, the person grasped the addiction in an attempt to nurture life, spirit, and the Self in the process of chasing perfection. Many recovering addicts firmly grasp the spiritual aspect of recovery because most are extremely grateful to have such a precious gift returned: the Self, a spiritual awareness, and the ability to connect with others in a meaningful, nurturing way."

2.84 Yong, J, Kim J, Han S.S, and Puchalski C.M. (2008, Winter). **Development and validation of a scale assessing spiritual needs for Korean patients with cancer.** *J Palliat Care.* 24(4):240-6.

Spiritual Need Scale (SNS). Yong et al.

"Relationship with God

Religious Needs

Meaning and Purpose

Existentialistic Needs (Reflection/Meaning)

 Acceptance of Dying

Hope and Peace

Need for Inner Peace

Love and Connection

Actively Giving."

This concludes the description of the eight spiritual disorders. They are presented not as condemnations, but as avenues of hope on which we can find relieve from our brokenness. The next section features various possibilities for that healing. We can learn to move away from our spiritual disorders.

3. Without Spiritual Disorder

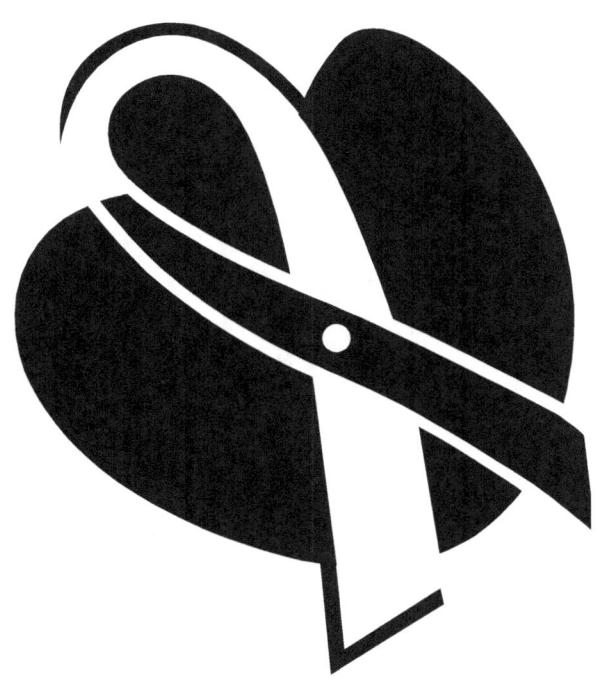

We have to understand spiritual disorders in order to comprehend spiritual order. The field of spiritual order is far wider than that of physical or mental order. It is determent mainly by organized religion for it is religious institutions, that generally set acceptable spiritual behavior. But spirituality goes beyond religions and includes all our relationships to God, a higher power, and the supernatural.

The diagnosis of a spiritual disorder is only the first step in this process. Other steps include, among others, methodologies of help, planning, implementation of help, and evaluation of outcomes. The categories of spiritual order and disorder are given as continuums, ranging from very good spiritual health on the left side to very harmful spiritual disorders on the right side.

The purpose of diagnosing spiritual disorders is to help people deal with them and to avoid any harm that may come because of their manifestation.

Most people want to be free from all disorders, be they physical, mental, or spiritual disorders. In the end, the physical disorders take over completely and we lose our lives. Spiritual disorders affect our physical and mental lives and hinder us as we try to cope with the issues around us.

Joylessness (SD1) robs us of our ability to live peacefully and fully in the face of the normal difficulties of life. On the other hand, joy strengthens us as we deal with problems.

110

Nothing is as destructive as self-centeredness (SD2) and selfishness. It robs us of our ability to serve, to help, or to bring others into our lives. It excludes God from our life, for God does not take second or third place. To live effective spiritual lives, we have to consider making God first, for He is the Creator and knows all about the world and us.

Much of our current culture is based on pleasure seeking (SD4). Nevertheless, with time, this too becomes boring and ineffective to bring us satisfaction. The whole world of entertainment in all its forms tries to bring pleasure into the lives of others. Entertainment has expanded in the area of news, religion, and education.

One of the greatest gifts we can receive is peace of mind, and knowing that the important things in life have been satisfied. Fear (SD5) and anxiety upset us and limit our joys. One of the greatest fears is that of the unknown. However, with some effort, we can search out answers to many questions.

We live in an age where many people have trouble telling right from wrong. Dishonesty (SD7) is rampant. It is hard to trust people who should be trustworthy. The range of dishonesty goes all the way from small deceptions to serious criminal behavior. However, all affect negatively both the performer of the dishonesty and the recipient.

There is a whole group of people who have written off their spiritual life because of some experience they had with a few people. We associate spirituality with religion. In addition, when religious people act hypocritically and unloving, people are disappointed, and often through the baby out with the wash-water. In many ways, spirituality is independent of religion.

The next four sections deal with the reduction or elimination of spiritual disorders. It is not enough to diagnose spiritual disorders; the key here is to deal with them positively.

Many physical diseases cannot be eliminated, so physicians and others try to reduce the harmful symptoms. That is not a solution to the problem, but it is often the best health care professionals can give. When I recently had a bad cold, I took an over-the-counter medication that reduced the symptoms and thus helped my body to heal itself. In a similar way, the section on fixing spiritual problems suggests many small ways to reduce the harm caused.

Following that section are three discussion guides that deal with more systemic changes toward better spiritual health. The first one is based on ethics sources, the other two on faith sources. The first faith source deals with help in specific spiritual disorders, the second source deals with general faith problems.

In a way, the cause of every kind of spiritual disorder is similar, namely wrong choices. Therefore the reader may want to deal with that problem and change to a lifestyle that will support good choices and good spiritual health. He may choose to live by faith and a clear purpose, rather than by the emotions of the moment.

3.1 Fixing Spiritual Disorders

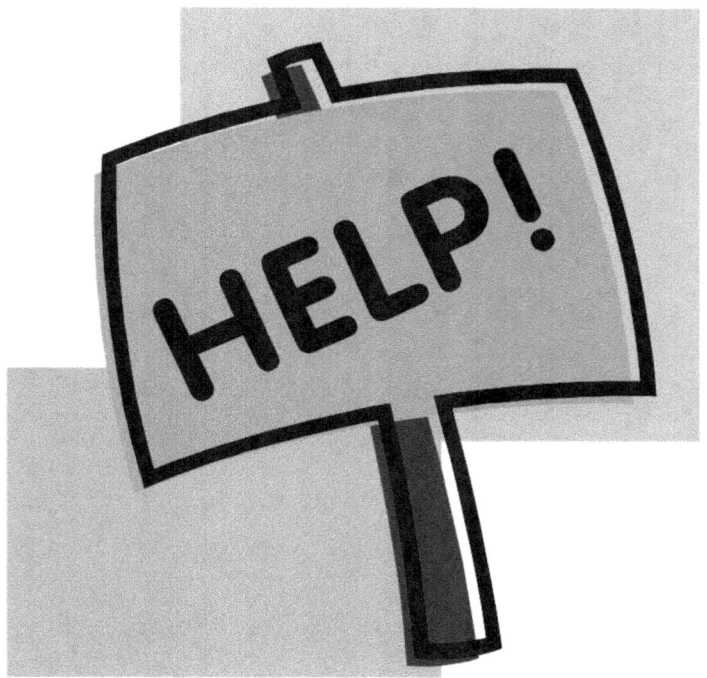

Spiritual disorders may be treated in at least two ways, which is in fixing them or healing them. In fixing spiritual disorders, the spiritual caregiver brings all behavioral and social science remedies to the situation. These include among others counseling, education, exercises, and group therapy.

Behavioral and social sciences treat the behaviors associated with the disorders, not the underlying causes. In that, they fix part of the disorder but do not touch their source.

Many methods used in medicine, health, religion, and social work may be helpful in that. The DSM does not provide treatment methods for the mental disorders. This volume, the SD1-8, does not attempt to present a complete listing or description of available methods.

In this section, only a brief presentation of possible remedies is given. Spiritual care has an extensive literature,

Reinhold Niebuhr's Prayer

"God, give me the serenity to accept the things I cannot change; the courage to change the things I can; and the wisdom to know the difference."

Prayer of St Francis modified by Charles C. Wise

"Lord, Make me an instrument of your health: where there is sickness, let me bring cure; where s injury, aid; where there is suffering, ease; where there is sadness comfort; where there is despair hope; where there is death, acceptance and peace Grant that I may not: So much seek to be justified, as to console; To obey as to understand; To be honored as to love For it is in giving of ourselves that we heal, It is in listening that we comfort, and in dying that we are born to eternal life."

3.11 How Best to Treat Spiritual Disorders?

In treating mental and spiritual disorders, we may focus on the symptoms of the person and deal with them directly. Paul McHugh and Phillip Slavney of Johns Hopkins University feel that the DSM is based on this approach. They are critical of this method and consider it a top-down approach.

Sigmund Freud developed this approach in psychoanalysis, a theory of human mental phenomena and behavior focusing on the influence of unconscious forces on the mental state.

The second approach is to deal with the problems from a larger perspective and add to the symptoms a focus on personality dimensions, motivated behavior and life encounters. In this approach, the patient's history is more important than the diagnosis. Hippocrates once wrote, "The natural healing force within each one of us is the greatest force in getting well." McHugh and Slavney prefer this bottom-up approach to diagnosis based on detailed life histories and an examination of the mental status.

Adolf Meyers developed this theory of psychobiology that focused on the whole person. This volume also rejects dualism of body and mind and deals with the whole person. It accepts the evidence-based approach rather than the naturopathic, homeopathic or chiropractic one.

3.12 Monod S, Brennan M, Rochat E, Martin E, Rochat S, Büla C. J. (2011, November). **Instruments measuring spirituality in clinical research: a systematic review.** *J Gen Intern Med.* 26(11):1345-57.

Abstract Introduction: "This study's aims were to identify instruments used in clinical research that measure spirituality; to propose a classification of these instruments; and to identify those instruments that could provide information on the need for spiritual intervention."

Methods: "A systematic literature search in MEDLINE, CINHAL, PsycINFO, ATLA, and EMBASE databases, using the terms "spirituality" and "adults," and limited to journal articles was performed to identify clinical studies that used a spiritual assessment instrument."

Results: "Thirty-five instruments were retrieved and classified into measures of general spirituality (N = 22), spiritual well-being (N = 5), spiritual coping (N = 4), and spiritual needs (N = 4) according to the conceptual classification. Instruments most frequently used in clinical research were the FACIT-Sp and the Spiritual Well-Being Scale."

Conclusions: "Instruments identified in this systematic review assess multiple dimensions of spirituality, and the proposed classifications should help clinical researchers interested in investigating the complex relationship between spirituality and health. Findings underscore the scarcity of instruments specifically designed to measure a patient's current spiritual state."

3.13 Basic Interventions

This section outlines areas of intervention but does not go into details. The literature of the spiritual-related professions is extensive and available to those working on spiritual interventions.

a. Intentional Ministry of Presence. Just the sympathetic presence of a spiritual caregiver is at times very helpful. Many spiritual visits last just ten minutes and are effective in refocusing spiritual problems.

b. Meaning Making. Life has to have meaning. By focusing on the meaning of events, spiritual caregivers often open up many helpful resources.

c. Grief Work. Grief often floods people and they are unable see their way out. By going through the grief process (denial, anger, bargaining. depression, acceptance), they can be freed from these limitations.

d. Clinical Use of Prayer. Prayer often opens up areas of concern that were tightly locked up. Talking to God brings to the situation resources that can be very helpful.

e. Confession – Guilt. Talking about a spiritual problem with a counselor, pastor or God is often helpful.

f. Forgiveness Work. There is a place for going through the steps of forgiveness (acknowledging anger, giving up revenge, offender's perspective, accepting hurt, extending compassion) and freeing oneself of the burdens that bind.

g. Thanking. Just learning to be thankful can be a major way to restore a healthy spiritual life. Thankfulness focuses on the ultimate giver, who for spiritual people is God.

h. Life Review – Spiritual Autobiography. By reviewing the blessings of life, you see things from a larger perspective. Many of the smaller problems lose their significance and the important things stand out.

i. Scripture Education. The Bible is a good textbook for learning order and disorder. It contains much good counsel and many case studies of people with spiritual disorders and ways how they overcame them.

j. Reframing God Assumptions. Since spirituality deals with our relationship with God, we have to know who God is. Often we assume we know, when in reality we are not sure. . Examining these assumptions may be helpful in our spiritual growth.

k. Encouraging Connection with a Spiritual Community. We grow spiritually as we talk with others about spiritual things. We learn what works and what does not.

l. Creative Writing. Writing out our story helps us examine and organize our thinking. Thus we are forced to face our spiritual live and examine it. Write a journal.

3.14 Spiritual Assessment Questions.

Touro Institute, **Spiritual Assessment and Care**, Retrieved http://www.touroinstitute.com/6%20Spiritual%20Assessment %20and%20Care.pdf (2012, December).

a. – "What do I believe in?

b. – What gives my life meaning?

c. – What makes me smile?

d. – What is my favorite part of creation?

e. – If I could be anywhere, where would I be?

f. – What do I hope for?

g. – Who do I love and who loves me?

h. – When do I feel most connected to others?

i. – What is my understanding of spirituality?

j. – How do I express my spirituality?

k. – What relationship do I have with a higher being?

l. – Why is spiritual care important to me?

m. – What spiritual rituals are meaningful to me?"

3.15 Visual Rehearsing

One way to deal with specific spiritual disorders is to focus on the possible potential order in our lives. Dwelling on disorder results in more disorder. Concentrating and rehearsing order leads towards order.

This is similar to Dr. Barry Krakow's Imagery Rehearsal Therapy, where participants learn how to free themselves from self-selected nightmares. They record the nightmare and write it down as a positive dream imagery. Afterward, each participant uses imagery to rehearse her own "new dream" scenario for 10 to 15 minutes. Next she describes her old nightmare, and how she changed it. After this, participants are encouraged to establish the process mentally. They are instructed to rehearse a new dream for at least 5 to 20 minutes each day.

As a person who strives to live a healthy spiritual life, I realize that spiritual persons are just as real as physical ones. The Creator is here and real long before He created the real trees and men that we see today around us. God produced us. We are His product. He is not just in our imagination, He is here as a person in reality. My grandfather, whom I never met, was real, even while I never saw him in life. I am his product. Our imagination can help us visualize God, but we do not depend on visualization to know that God is real.

By painting mind pictures of the things of God we can focus on the beauty and strength of the order that God so freely provides. The negative drops off, the positive takes over.

3.16 Light Therapy

In some places, February lacks sunny weather. I noticed that first while teaching at Andrews University in Michigan. To cheer up the students, the university provided a day off in February that they called ski-day. Moreover, many of us went skiing and returned happier.

It has been known for a long time that prolonged cloudy weather contributes to depression and other mood disorders. Is it possible then that sunny weather and sunshine helps in the healing of spiritual disorders?

I read that God is light, and that darkness is associated with difficulties and harm. More crimes are committed at night than at daytime. Most of us shut down and sleep at night, and work during daytime. Many who have to work at night find that work difficult.

Dr. Karl Deisseroth, a researcher of optogenetics at the Stanford University's Clark Center, has been able to implant harmless light-sensitive viruses into neurons of mice, and with strong yellow light was able to turn off the cocaine addiction of cocaine- addicted mice. A similar procedure is also being explored with depression, anxiety, and migraines.

Light therapy consists of exposure to specific wavelengths of light. It is used in the treatment of skin disorders, sleep disorder and some psychiatric disorders. Further research may show that it may be useful with spiritual disorders.

3.17 As I Think, so I Feel and Do

I am struggling with my computer software. It does not want to work for me. I feel discouraged. It is time for me to help my wife, but I cannot do that. When I think failure, I feel my distress, and center my life on my pain.

On the other hand, when I think of my blessings, I feel on top of the world, and sing.

The think-feel-do model teaches me to think positively, to feel the joy of living, and to serve others in need. It all starts with my thinking.

Abstract. "Developed by two master clinicians Dennis Greenberger and Christine Padesky with extensive experience in cognitive therapy treatment and training, *Mind Over Mood: Change How You Feel by Changing the Way You Think (The Guilford Press,* 1995, New York*)* shows readers how to improve their lives using cognitive therapy. The book is designed to be used alone or in conjunction with professional treatment. Step-by-step worksheets teach specific skills that have helped hundreds and thousands of people conquer depression, panic attacks, anxiety, anger, guilt, shame, low self-esteem, eating disorders, substance abuse and relationship problems. Readers learn to use mood questionnaires to identify, rate, and track changes in feelings; change the thoughts that contribute to problems; follow step-by-step strategies to improve moods; and take action to improve daily living and relationships."

3.2 Ethics Discussion Guides

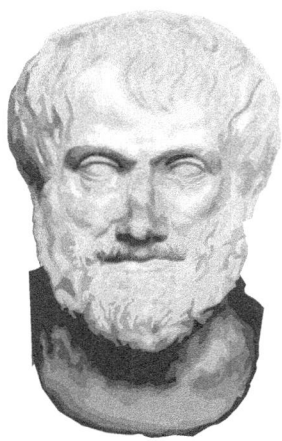

In Part One of this volume, I presented an introduction to spiritual order and disorder. In Part Two, I described the eight spiritual disorders in a way that may be useful for a diagnosis of these disorders. Now Part Three deals with the fixing and healing of spiritual disorders.

There are at least three approaches to the healing of spiritual disorders. One of them is a behavioral science research approach. That approach was used in Parts One and Two.

Then there is the ethical approach. Ethics, also known as moral philosophy, here deals with the concepts of right and wrong, with order and disorder. According to Aristotle (pictured above), when a person acts in harmony with his nature, and realizes his full potential, he will do well and be content.

3.21 Aristotle on the Ethics of Joy. SD1

Read the quotations and discuss the questions:

"With those who identify happiness with virtue, our account is in harmony; for to virtue belongs virtuous activity. But it makes, perhaps, no small difference whether we place the **chief good** in possession or in **use**, in state of mind or in **activity.** For the state of mind may exist without producing any good result, as in a man who is asleep or in some other way quite inactive, but the activity cannot; for one who has the activity will of necessity be acting, and acting well. And as in the Olympic Games it is not the most beautiful and the strongest that are crowned but those who compete (for it is some of these that are victorious), so those who act win, and rightly win, the noble and good things in life."

Question 1. Why is activity the chief good? _____

"Their life is also in itself pleasant. For **pleasure is a state of soul,** and to each man that which he is said to be a lover of is pleasant; e.g. not only is a horse pleasant to the lover of horses, and a spectacle to the lover of sights, but also in the same way just acts are pleasant to the lover of justice and in general virtuous acts to the lover of virtue."

Q2. What is pleasure? Answer 2: **A state of mind we choose.**

"Now for most men their **pleasures are in conflict** with one another because these are **not by nature pleasant**, but the lovers of what is noble find pleasant the things that are by nature pleasant; and virtuous actions are such, so that these are pleasant for such men as well as in their own nature."

Q3. Why are pleasures often in conflict? _____

"Their life, therefore, has no further need of pleasure as a sort of adventitious charm, but has its pleasure in itself. For, besides what we have said, **the man who does not rejoice in noble actions is not even good**; since no one would call a man just who did not enjoy acting justly, nor any man liberal who did not enjoy liberal actions; and similarly in all other cases. If this is so, **virtuous actions must be in themselves pleasant.** But they are also good and noble, and have each of these attributes in the highest degree, since the good man judges well about these attributes; his judgment is such as we have described. **Happiness then is the best, noblest, and most pleasant thing in the world**, and these attributes are not severed as in the inscription at Delos-

'Most noble is that which is most just, and best is health; but pleasantest is it to win what we love.'

For all these properties belong to the best activities; and these, or one- the best- of these, we identify with happiness."

Q4. Why are virtuous acts pleasant? _____

Aristotle, **Nicomachean Ethics**, 350 BC, I-8.

3.22   Aristotle on Kindness and Self-centeredness. SD2

"To take Kindness next: the definition of it will show us towards whom it is felt, why, and in what frames of mind. Kindness-under the influence of which a man is said to 'be kind' may be defined as **helpfulness towards someone in need,** not in return for anything, nor for the advantage of the helper himself, but for that of the person helped."

Q1. How do kindness, help, and need relate? _____

"**Kindness** is great if shown to one who is in **great need,** or who needs what is important and hard to get, or who needs it at an important and difficult crisis; or if the helper is the only, the first, or the chief person to give the help."

Q2. What is great kindness? _____

"Hence those who stand by us in **poverty** or in banishment, even if they do not help us much, **are yet really kind to us, because our need is great** and the occasion pressing; for instance, the man who gave the mat in the Lyceum. The helpfulness must therefore meet, preferably, just this kind of need; and failing just this kind, some other kind as great or greater. We now see to whom, why, and under what conditions kindness is shown; and these facts must form the basis of our arguments."

Q3.Why is help in poverty so important ? _____

126

"We must show that the persons helped are, or have been, in such pain and need as has been described, and that their helpers gave, or are giving, the kind of help described, in the kind of need described. We can also see how to eliminate the idea of **kindness and make our opponents appear unkind**: we may maintain that they are being or have been helpful simply to promote their own interest-this, as has been stated, is not kindness; or that **their action was accidental**, or was **forced** upon them; or that they were not doing a favor, but merely **returning** one, whether they know this or not-in either case the action is a mere return, and is therefore not a kindness even if the doer does not know how the case stands."

Q4. What marks unkind acts? _____

"In considering this subject we must look at all the categories: an act may be an **act of kindness** because (1) it is a particular thing, (2) it has a particular magnitude, or (3) quality, or (4) is done at a particular time, or (5) place. As evidence of the want of kindness, we may point out that a smaller service had been refused to the man in need; or that the same service, or an equal or greater one, has been given to his enemies; these facts show that **the service in question was not done for the sake of the person helped**. Or we may point out that the thing desired was **worthless** and that the helper knew it: no one will admit that he is in need of what is worthless."

Q5. What makes an act a kindness? _____

Aristotle, **Rhetoric** (350 BC) II:7.

3.23 C. Joybell C on Materialism. SD3

"The shame and the **downfall of a modern materialistic** society is **her inabilities** to treasure, care for, admire, adore, cherish, value, revere, respect, uphold, uplift, protect, shield, defend, safeguard, treasure, and **love her children**.

Q1. What is the problem of materialistic society? _____

"I praise all the cultures of this world that naturally harbor and actively manifest these instincts. If a nation or if a population of people **fails to recognize the excellent value** and distinction of the lives of her **children** and is defective enough to have lost the capability of expressing and acting upon these instincts then there is **nothing that can save that nation** or those people."

Q2. What excellent values do children have? _____

"The **prosperity of a people is not measured in banks**, financial markets, economy and the death of its humanity is evident not through the loss of life but in the loss of love for its children."

Q3. What measures prosperity?_____

C. JoyBell C. <http://cjoybellc.com> (2012 October).

3.24   Aristotle on Desires and Pleasure-seeking. SD4

"I count him **braver** who overcomes his **desires** than him who conquers his enemies; for the hardest victory is over self."

"He who is to be a good ruler must have first been ruled."

"Different men seek after happiness in different ways and by different means, and so make for themselves **different modes** of life and forms of government."

"Bring your **desires** down to your present means. Increase them only when your increased means permit."

"To enjoy the things we ought and to hate the things we ought to have the greatest bearing on excellence of **character**."

"**Virtue of character** is concerned with pleasures and pains. For it is pleasure that causes us to do base actions, and pain that causes us to abstain from fine ones. Hence we need to have had the appropriate upbringing—right from early youth, as Plato says—to make us find enjoyment or pain in the right things; for this is the correct education." Aristotle, **Nicomachean Ethics,** 11049-13

Q1. With what quotations do you agree and why? _____

Q2. With what quotations do you disagree and why? _____

3.25 Aristotle on Fear. SD5

"Plainly the things we fear are terrible things, and these are, to speak without qualification, evils; for which reason people even define **fear as expectation of evil.** Now we fear all evils, e.g. disgrace, poverty, disease, friendlessness, death, but the brave man is not thought to be concerned with all; for **to fear some things is even right** and noble, and it is base not to fear them- e.g. **disgrace**; he who fears this is good and modest, and he who does not is shameless."

Q1. When is it good to fear? _____

"Poverty and disease we perhaps ought **not to fear**, nor in general the things that **do not proceed from vice** and are not due to a man himself."

Q2. Why should we not fear disease? _____

"But not even the man who is fearless of these is **brave**. Yet we apply the word to him also in virtue of a similarity; for some who in the dangers of war are cowards are liberal and are confident in face of the loss of money."

"Nor is a man a coward if he fears insult to his wife and children or envy or anything of the kind; nor **brave** if he is confident when he is about to be flogged. With what sort of terrible things, then, is the **brave** man concerned?"

Q3. With what is the brave man concerned? _____

"Surely with the greatest; for no one is more likely than he to stand his ground against what is awe-inspiring. Now **death** is the most terrible of all things; for it is the end, **and nothing is thought to be any longer either good or bad for the dead.** But the brave man would not seem to be concerned even with death in all circumstances, e.g. at sea or in disease. In what circumstances, then? Surely in the noblest. Now such deaths are those in battle; for these take place in the greatest and noblest danger. And these are correspondingly honored in city-states and at the courts of monarchs. Properly, then, he will be called brave who is **fearless in face of a noble death,** and of all **emergencies that involve death**; and the emergencies of war are in the highest degree of this kind."

Q4. Do we have to fear death? _____

"Yet at sea also, and in disease, **the brave man is fearless,** but not in the same way as the seaman; for he has **given up hope of safety**, and dislikes the thought of death in this shape, while **they are hopeful** because of their experience."

Q5. How does hope relate to fear? _____

"At the same time, we show courage in situations where there is the opportunity of showing prowess or where death is noble; but in these forms of death neither of these conditions is fulfilled."

Aristotle, **Nicomachean Ethics**, 350 BC, III:6.

3.26 Orson Scott Card on Forgiveness. SD6

"**A Great Rabbi** stands, teaching in the marketplace. It happens that a husband finds proof that morning of his wife's adultery, and a mob carries her to the marketplace to stone her to death. There is a familiar version of this story, but a friend of mine - a Speaker for the Dead - has told me of two other Rabbis that faced the same situation. Those are the ones I'm going to tell you."

"The Rabbi walks forward and stands beside the woman. Out of respect for him, the mob forbears and waits with the stones heavy in their hands. 'Is there any man here,' he says to them, 'who has not desired another man's wife, another woman's husband?' They murmur and say, 'We all know the desire, but Rabbi **none of us has acted on it**.'"

"The Rabbi says, 'Then kneel down and give thanks that God has made you strong.' He takes the woman by the hand and leads her out of the market. Just before he lets her go, he whispers to her, 'Tell the Lord Magistrate who saved his mistress, and then he'll know I am his loyal servant.' So the **woman lives** because the community is too corrupt to protect itself from disorder."

Q1. Was that a good reason to forgive her? _____

"**Another Rabbi. Another city.** He goes to her, stops the mob as in the other story, and says, 'Which of you is without sin? Let him cast the first stone.'"

132

"The people are abashed, and they forget their unity of purpose in the memory of their own individual sins. ' Someday,' they think, 'I may be like this woman. In addition, I will hope for forgiveness and another chance. I should treat her as I wish to be treated.'"

"As they opened their hands and let their stones fall to the ground, the Rabbi picks up one of the fallen stones, lifts it high over the woman's head and throws it straight down with all his might it crushes her skull and dashes her brain among the cobblestones. ' Nor am I without sins,' he says to the people, 'but if we allow only perfect people to enforce the law, the law will soon be dead – and our city with it.'"

"So **the woman died** because her community was too rigid to endure her deviance."

"The famous version of this story is noteworthy because it is so startlingly rare in our experience. Most communities lurch between decay and rigor mortis and when they veer too far they die. Only one Rabbi dared to expect of us such a perfect balance that we could preserve the law and still forgive the deviation. So of course, **we killed him.**"

Q2. Whom did we kill? Why? _____

-San Angelo, Letters **to an Incipient Heretic**, Orson Scott Card, **Speaker for the Dead.** < www.orsonscottcard.com/>

3.27 Anthony Trollope on Dishonesty. SD7

"Nevertheless a certain class of dishonesty, **dishonesty magnificent in its proportions, and climbing into high places,** has become at the same time so rampant and so splendid that there seems to be reason for fearing that men and women will be taught to feel that **dishonesty, if it can become splendid, will cease to be abominable.** If dishonesty can live in a gorgeous palace with pictures on all its walls, and gems in all its cupboards, with marble and ivory in all its corners, and can give Apician dinners, and get into Parliament, and deal in millions, then dishonesty is not disgraceful, and the man dishonest after such a fashion is not a low scoundrel."

Q1. How is dishonesty rampant today? _____

"Instigated, I say, by some such reflections as these, I sat down in my new house to write The Way We Live Now. And as I had ventured to take the whip of the satirist into my hand, I went beyond the iniquities of the great speculator who robs everybody, and made an onslaught also on other vices;--on the intrigues of girls who want to get married, on the luxury of young men who prefer to remain single, and on the puffing propensities of authors who desire to **cheat** the public into buying their volumes."

Q2. Who today cheats regularly? _____

"It is a lamentable fact that men and women lend themselves to these practices that are neither vindictive nor ordinarily dishonest. It has become **"the custom of the trade**," under the veil of which excuse so many tradesmen justify their malpractices! When a struggling author learns that so much has been done for A by the Barsetshire Gazette, so much for B by the Dillsborough Herald, and, again, so much for C by that powerful metropolitan organ the Evening Pulpit, and is told also that A and B and C have been favored through personal interest, he also goes to work among the editors, or the editors' wives,--or perhaps, if he cannot reach their wives, with their wives' first or second cousins. When once the feeling has come upon an editor or a critic that he may allow himself to be influenced by other considerations than the duty he owes to the public, all sense of critical or of editorial honesty falls from him at once. Facilis descensus Averni. In a very short time, that editorial honesty becomes ridiculous to him. It is for other purpose that he wields the power; and when he is told what his duty is, and what should be his conduct, the preacher of such doctrine seems to him to be quixotic. "Where have you lived, my friend, for the last twenty years," he says in spirit, if not in word, "that you come out now with such stuff as old-fashioned as this?" And thus, **dishonesty begets dishonesty, until dishonesty seems to be beautiful**. How nice to be good-natured! How glorious to assist struggling young authors, especially if the young author be also a pretty woman! How gracious to oblige a friend! Then the motive, though still pleasing, departs further from the border of what is good.

Trollope, Anthony. **Autobiography of Anthony Trollope** < www.anthonytrollope.com/> (2012, October)

Q3. How does editorial honesty apply in other fields? _____

3.28 Aristotle on Wisdom. SD8

"The **wise man** does not expose himself needlessly to danger, since there are few things for which he cares sufficiently; but he is willing, in great crises, to give even his life--knowing that under certain conditions it is not worthwhile to live. He is of a disposition **to do men service**, though he is ashamed to have a service done to him."

Q1. Why is it wise to serve? _____

"To confer a kindness is a mark of **superiority**; to receive one is a mark of **subordination**... He does not take part in public displays... He is open in his dislikes and preferences; he talks and acts frankly, because of his contempt for men and things... He is never fired with admiration, since there is nothing great in his eyes. He cannot live in complaisance with others, except it be a friend; complaisance is the characteristic of a slave... He never feels malice, and always forgets and passes over injuries... He is not fond of talking... It is no concern of his that he should be praised, or that others should be blamed. He does not speak evil of others, even of his enemies, unless it is to them."

Q2. Where do you disagree with Aristotle? _____

Q3. What would you add as a sign of wisdom? _____

Aristotle, **Ethics,** 350 BC.

3.3 Faith Discussion Guides

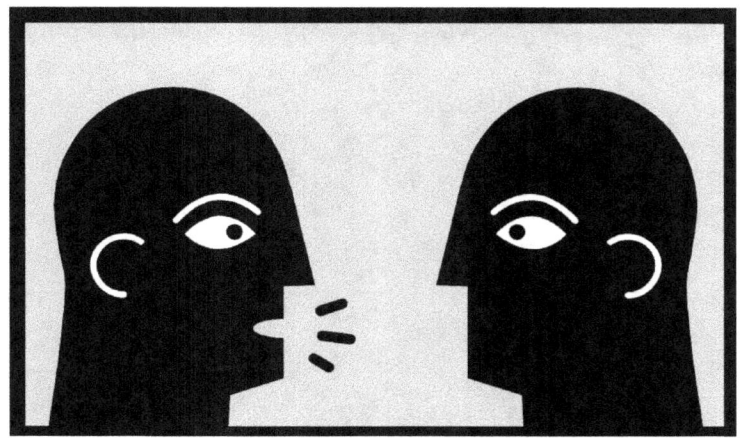

Specific interventions may help with spiritual disorders, but only a fully focused spiritual lifestyle can bring healing to the individual.

That lifestyle should be based on an acceptance of a higher power in one's life, and on a loving relationship with God and others.

God is the creator who has given us physical bodies and minds to control them and the world around us. Wherever we go, we are subject to the order he has established. When we violate that order, we reap spiritual disorders.

When we try to follow his order, all areas of life support all others. There is a healing that goes beyond the physical, the mental, or the spiritual and affects all three. In some way, these three are not separate, but just different perspectives of a person.

We are very blessed when we learn to live without spiritual disorders. Whatever our circumstances, we gain strength from knowing that we have a partner who can see us through.

Healing spiritual disorders is a process that requires a healer, a person to be healed, and a disorder from which the person is to be healed. If one of the three is missing, there can be no healing.

God is the creator and the healer. The important thing is not the dates of specific creations, but the fact that God made everything. Many people are hung up on the dates for creation. The Bible, nor any other writing, gives the exact dates for creation of the universe, the world, or of life. In creation, God made everything, in healing God restores everything to its original order. Only as we acknowledge that we have a disorder can we be healed. Without that, there can be no healing. That is why the diagnosis of spiritual disorders is fundamental to the healing process.

There follow a number of discussion guides that are based on selected Bible passages. People throughout the ages have struggled with spiritual disorders and have found answers in various writings. Here we use the Bible primarily as a source of learning specific ways to deal with spiritual disorders.

3.31 Paul on Joylessness: SD1

"Philippians 1:4 Always in every prayer of mine making **request for you all with joy**, 1:25 and being confident of this, I know that I shall remain and continue with you all for your progress and **joy of faith.**"

"2:2 **Fulfill my joy** by being like-minded, having the same love, being of one accord, of one mind. 4:1 Therefore, my beloved and longed-for brethren, **my joy** and crown, so stand fast in the Lord, beloved. 1:18 What then? Only that in every way, whether in pretense or in truth, Christ is preached; and **in this I rejoice, yes, and will rejoice.**"

"2:16 Holding fast the word of life, so that **I may rejoice** in the day of Christ that I have not run in vain or labored in vain. 2:17 Yes, and if I am being poured out as a drink offering on the sacrifice and service of your faith, **I am glad and rejoice** with you all. 2:18 For the same reason you also **be glad and rejoice with me.** 2:28 Therefore I sent him the more eagerly, that when you see him again **you may rejoice.**"

"3:1 Finally, my brethren, **rejoice in the Lord**. For me to write the same things to you is not tedious, but for you it is safe. 3:3 For we are the circumcision, who worship God in the Spirit, **rejoice in Christ Jesus.**"

"4:4 Rejoice **in the Lord** always. Again I will say, **rejoice**! 4:10 **I rejoice in the Lord** greatly, your care of me has flourished." Philippians 1-4

Discuss and answer the following questions.

Q1. How do you pray in joy? _____

Q2. What is the joy of faith? _____

Q3. How can others fulfill my joy?   A3. **Being like-minded**

Q4. How are Paul's brothers his joy? _____

Q5. In what does Paul rejoice? _____

Q6. How will Paul rejoice in the day of Christ? _____

Q7. How do we rejoice in the return of friends? _____

Q8. How can I rejoice in the Lord? _____

Q9. Can I rejoice in the Lord always? _____

Q10. What is the connection between caring and rejoicing? __

Q11. How can I walk spiritually in joy? _____

Q12. How do we worship God? A12. **In the Spirit**_____

3.32 Job on Self-centeredness: SD2

We are to be altruistic and put God and others first. Job, at the end of his book, summarized that well.

16 "If I have denied the desires of the **poor** or let the eyes of the widow grow weary,"

"17 **If** I have kept my bread **to myself**, not sharing it with the fatherless-"

"18 but from my youth I reared him as would a father, and from my birth I guided the widow-"

Q1. How do I keep my bread to myself? _____

"19 **if** I have seen anyone perishing for **lack** of clothing, or a **needy man** without a garment,"

"20 and his heart did not bless me for **warming him with the fleece** from my sheep,"

"21 **if** I have **raised my hand against** the fatherless, knowing that I had influence in court, 22 then let my arm fall from the shoulder, let it be broken off at the joint." Job 31:16-22

Q2. How do I help the needy? _____

Q3. How are Job's cases examples of unselfishness? _____

3.33 Paul on Materialism: SD3

Paul gave some good advice to his young friend Timothy:

"6 But godliness **with contentment** is great gain."

"7 For we brought **nothing** into this world, and it is certain we can carry nothing out."

"8 And having food and raiment let us be therewith **content**."

"9 But they that will be rich fall into temptation and a snare, and into many foolish and hurtful lusts, which drown men in **destruction** and perdition."

"10 For the **love of money** is the root of all evil: which while some coveted after, they have erred from the faith, and pierced themselves through with many sorrows."

"11 But you, O man of God, flee these things; and follow after righteousness, godliness, faith, **love**, patience, meekness."

"17 Charge them that are rich in this world, that they be not **high-minded**, nor trust in uncertain riches, but in the living God, who gives us richly all things to enjoy;"

"18 That they do good, that they be rich in good works, ready to **distribute**, willing to communicate." 1 Tim 6:6-11, 17, 18

Q1. Why should we not be materialistic? _____

3.34 Solomon on Pleasure-seeking. SD4

King Solomon in the book of Ecclesiastes tested to see if pleasure seeking would satisfy him.

"1 I said in mine heart, Go to now, I will prove thee with mirth, therefore enjoy pleasure: and, behold, this also is vanity. 2 I said of laughter, It is mad: and of mirth, what doeth it? 3 I sought in mine heart to give myself unto wine, yet acquainting mine heart with wisdom; and to lay hold on folly, till I might see what was that good for the sons of men, which they should do under the heaven all the days of their life."

"4 I made me great works; I build me houses; I planted me vineyards: 5 I made me gardens and orchards, and I planted trees in them of all kind of fruits: 6 I made me pools of water, to water therewith the wood that bring forth trees:"

"9 So I was great, and increased more than all that were before me in Jerusalem: also my wisdom remained with me. 10 And whatsoever mine eyes desired I kept not from them, I withheld not my heart from any joy; for my heart rejoiced in all my labor: and this was my portion of all my labor."

"11 Then I looked on all the works that my hands had wrought, and on the labor that I had labored to do: and, behold, all was vanity and vexation of spirit, and there was no profit under the sun." Ecclesiastes 2:1-11

Q1. Why is pleasure seeking useless? _____

3.35 Matthew and Others on Fearfulness. SD5

"28 And fear not them which kill the body, but are not able to kill the soul: but rather fear him which is able to destroy both soul and body in hell. 29 Are not two sparrows sold for a farthing? and one of them shall not fall on the ground without your Father. 30 But the very hairs of your head are all numbered. 31 Fear ye not therefore, ye are of more value than many sparrows." Matthew 10:28-31

"Faith, which is trust, and fear are opposite poles. If a man has the one, he can scarcely have the other in vigorous operation. He that has his trust set upon God does not need to dread anything except the weakening or the paralyzing of that trust." ~ Alexander MacLaren

"Worry is a cycle of inefficient thoughts whirling around a center of fear." Corrie Ten Boom

"How strange this fear of death is! We are never frightened at a sunset." George Macdonald

"Fear of something is at the root of hate for others, and hate within will eventually destroy the hater." George Washington Carver

"Faith activates God – Fear activates the Enemy." Joel Osteen

Q1. How can we live without fear? _____

3.36 Luke on Unforgiveness. SD6

One of the best studies on forgiveness concerns the Prodigal Son, found in Luke 15:11-32. In accepting God's love, the father in the story took on God's forgiveness and then forgave his prodigal son. Discuss the reasons for the marked passages.

"11 And he said, a certain man had two sons: 12 and the younger of them said to his father, Father, give me the portion of goods that fall to me. And he divided unto them his living. 13 And not many days after the younger son gathered all together, and took his journey into a far country, and **there wasted his substance with riotous living."**

"14 And when he had spent all, there arose a mighty famine in that land; and he began to **be in want.**15 And he went and joined himself to a citizen of that country; and he sent him into his fields to feed swine. 16 And he would fain have filled his belly with the husks that the swine did eat: and no man gave unto him."

"17 And when he came to himself, he said, How many hired servants of my father's have bread enough and to spare, and I perish with hunger! 18 I will arise and go to my father, and will say unto him, Father**, I have sinned against heaven, and before thee,** 19 And am no more worthy to be called thy son: make me as one of thy hired servants."

"20 And he arose, and came to his father. But when he was yet a great way off, **his father saw him, and had compassion,** and ran, and fell on his neck, and kissed him. 21

And the son said unto him, Father, I have sinned against heaven, and in thy sight, and am no more worthy to be called your son."

"22 But the father said to his servants, Bring forth the best robe, and put it on him; and put a ring on his hand, and shoes on his feet: 23 And bring hither the fatted calf, and kill it; and let us eat, and be merry: 24 For this my son was dead, and is alive again; **he was lost, and is found (No revenge on the part of the father).** And they began to be merry."

"25 Now his elder son was in the field: and as he came and drew nigh to the house, he heard music and dancing. 26 And he called one of the servants, and asked what these things meant. 27 And he said unto him, Thy brother is come; and thy father hath killed the fatted calf, because he hath received him safe and sound. 28 And **he was angry (his unforgiveness lead to anger), and would not go in:** therefore came his father out to entreat him. 29 And he answering said to his father, Lo, these many years do I serve thee, neither transgressed I at any time thy commandment: and yet thou never gave me a kid, that I might make merry: 30 But as soon as this thy son was come, which hath devoured thy living with harlots, thou hast killed for him the fatted calf. 31 And he said unto him, Son, thou art ever with me, and all that I have is yours. 32 It was meet that we should make merry, and be glad: for this **your brother was dead, and is alive again;** and was lost, and is **found (and forgiven)."** Luke 15:11-32

Q1. How do you practice forgiveness? _____

146

3.37 Isaiah on Dishonesty. SD7

Isaiah lived about 1000 years before Christ, and was concerned with his self-centeredness (SD2), fear (SD5), and dishonesty (SD7). God healed him by forgiving him (SD6).

The Glory of God. "In the year that king Uzziah died I saw also the LORD sitting upon a throne, high and lifted up, and his train filled the temple. Above it stood the seraphims: each one had six wings; with twain he covered his face, and with twain he covered his feet, and with twain he did fly. And one cried unto another, and said, Holy, holy, holy, is the LORD of hosts: the whole earth is full of his glory. And the posts of the door moved at the voice of him that cried, and the house was filled with smoke."

Isaiah's Spiritual Disorder. "Then said I, Woe is me! for I am undone; because I am a man of unclean lips, and I dwell in the midst of a people of unclean lips (SD7): for mine eyes have seen the King, the LORD of hosts."

God's Spiritual Healing. "Then flew one of the seraphims unto me, having a live coal in his hand, which he had taken with the tongs from off the altar: And he laid it upon my mouth, and said, Lo, this hath touched thy lips; and your iniquity is taken away, and thy sin purged (SD6). Also I heard the voice of the Lord, saying, Whom shall I send, and who will go for us? Then said I, Here am I; send me." Isaiah 6: 1-6

Discuss and answer the following questions.

Q1. How does Isaiah describe God? _____

Q2. How is the earth full of the glory of God? _____

Q3. What made Isaiah recognize his dishonesty? _____

Q4. What are unclean lips? **A mouth that speaks deceit.**____

Q5. Who are the people of unclean lips? _____

Q6. How did seeing the King make him see his uncleanliness?

Q7. Did Isaiah request forgiveness? _____

Q8. Did the angel burn out Isaiah's dishonesty? _____

Q9. Is dishonesty a sin? _____

Q10. What did God ask from Isaiah? _____

Q11. Why did God make that request?

Q12. How did Isaiah respond? _____

Q13. How does your spiritual life make you honest? _____

3.38 Paul on Unspecified/Addiction. SD8

While there are other spiritual disorders that fall into this category, I chose thankfulness and thanklessness as good examples to consider here.

"1:3 **We give thanks to God and the Father** of our Lord Jesus Christ, praying always for you, 4 Since we heard of your faith in Christ Jesus, and of the love which ye have to all the saints,"

"1:12 **Giving thanks unto the Father**, which hath made us meet to be partakers of the inheritance of the saints in light:"

"2:6 As ye have therefore received Christ Jesus the Lord, so walk you in him: 7 Rooted and built up in him, and established in the faith, as ye have been taught, abounding therein with **thanksgiving."**

"3:15 And let the peace of Christ rule in your hearts, to which indeed you were called in one body. And **be thankful."**

"16 Let the word of Christ dwell in you richly, teaching and admonishing one another in all wisdom, singing psalms and hymns and spiritual songs, **with thankfulness in your hearts to God."**

"17 And whatever you do, in word or deed, do everything in the name of the Lord Jesus, **giving thanks to God the Father** through him." Col 1:3-4, 1:12, 2:6-7, 3:15-17

Q1. What does the Word of Christ teach us? _____

12 **"Blessed** is the man that **endures temptation**: for when he is tried, he shall receive the crown of life, which the Lord hath promised to them that love him."

"13 Let no man say when he is tempted, I am tempted of God: for God cannot be tempted with evil, neither tempts he any man:"

"14 But every man is tempted, when he is drawn away of his own lust, and enticed."

"15 Then when lust hath conceived, it brings forth sin: and sin, when it is finished, brings forth death."

"16 Do not err, my beloved brother."

"17 Every good **gift** and every perfect gift is from above, and comes down from the Father of lights, with whom is no variableness, neither shadow of turning." James 1: 12-17

"Submit yourselves therefore to God. Resist the devil, and he will flee from you." James 4:7

Q2. How are people tempted? _____

Q3. Where do our gifts come from? _____

3.4 Spiritual Discussion Guide

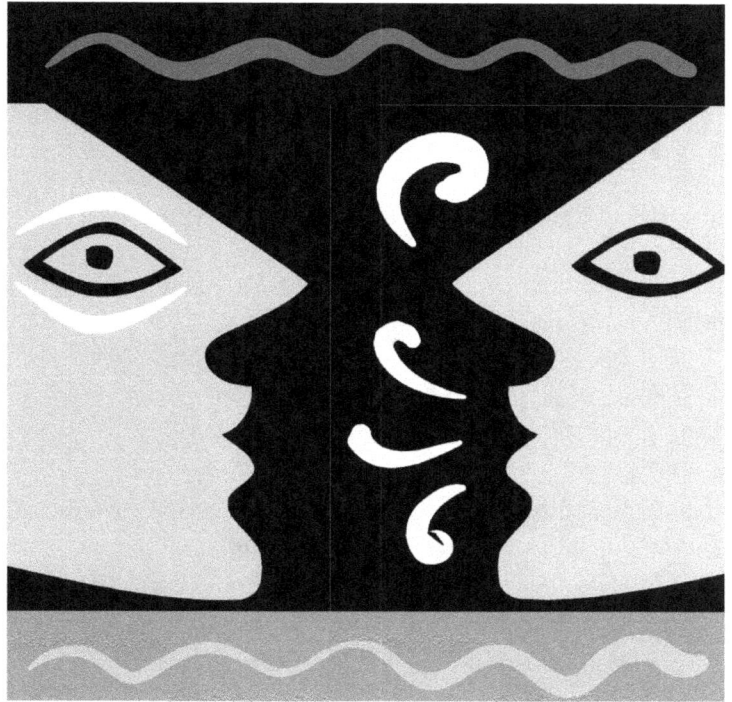

There are a number of Bible passages, that deal with all or most spiritual disorders. A study and application of them can help bring healing to the disorderly.

What follows are seven spiritual discussions based on Biblical passages. These discussions focus on all spiritual disorders identified in this volume, and not on one specific disorder, like in the previous section.

151

3.41 Spiritual Dangers

One of the best descriptions of people with spiritual disorders is found in the Bible in 2 Timothy 3:2-5. The number of the spiritual disorder, used in this volume, is given in brackets.

"2 For men will be lovers of themselves (SD2), lovers of money (SD3), boasters, proud (SD1), blasphemers, disobedient to parents, unthankful, unholy (SD5),"

"3 unloving, unforgiving, slanderers, without self-control, brutal, despisers of good (SD7),"

"4 traitors, headstrong, haughty (SD6), lovers of pleasure, rather than lovers of God (SD4),"

"5 having a form of godliness but denying its power. And from such people turn away! (SD8)" 2 Tim 3:2-5

2 Timothy 1:7, reads: "For God has not given us a spirit of fear (SD5) and timidity, but of power, love, and self-discipline."

All that is the opposite of lovers of God and goodness (SD2,1,7), of giving and service (SD3,4), of peace and forgiveness (SD5,6). They are forms of godlessness or spirituality that are ineffective to bring about spiritual healing.

Q1. What are examples of the three bad lovers? _____.

Q2. What are examples of the three good lovers? _____.

Lovers put a special emphasis on one aspect of their lives. They are controlled by the things or persons they love. We all are lovers of something or somebody. Being a lover of something is a spiritual characteristic, but not necessarily a positive one or a religious one. One or more of our spiritual disorders may be severe enough to affect all we do.

Q3. What is your main spiritual strength? _____.

A lover of God tries to listen to God and do his will. To him, the Bible is the Word of God. The Bible helps him establish his priorities. His own interests become secondary while God's remain primary.

Q4. How do you face these dangers? _____.

Q5. How does love overcome these dangers? _____.

Q6. How does God's power overcome these dangers? _____.

Spirituality can be powerful or powerless. If it is just a form, it is powerless to help the individual. For many individuals, spirituality is a habit or social activity that satisfies the minimum desires for the good life. If it is a deep inner life and a connection with God, it can give purpose to life and enrich all a person does.

Q7. What is the part of self-discipline in healing? _____.

Q8. What is the difference between form and effective love? _

3.42 Spiritual Love

We are to center our lives outside of self, not on self (SD2). That is one of the central teachings of Christ. Christ taught God-centered love. It is summarized below in the Bible by Matthew:

"Master, which is the great commandment in the law? Jesus said unto him, You shall love the Lord (SD2) your God with all your heart, and with all your soul, and with all your mind. This is the first and great commandment. And the second is like unto it, You shall love your neighbor (SD2) as yourself. On these two commandments hang all the law and the prophets." Matthew 22: 36-40

Christ in his Sermon on the Mountain presented the love remedy for human disorders:

"43 You have heard that it was said, 'You shall love your neighbor and hate your enemy.' 44 But I say to you, love your enemies (SD2), bless those who curse you (SD5), do good to those who hate you (SD7), and pray for **those who spitefully use you** (SD1) and persecute you (SD4), 45 that you may be sons of your Father in heaven (SD3); for He makes His sun rise on the evil and on the good (SD6), and sends rain on the just and on the unjust. 46 For if you love those who love you, what reward have you (SD4)? Do not even the tax collectors do the same? 47 And if you greet your brethren only, what do you do more than others? Do not even the tax collectors do so? 48 Therefore you shall be perfect, just as your Father in heaven is perfect." Matthew 5:43-48

The love of God is the ultimate greatest healing agent. The whole Bible as the Word of God is a textbook and casebook on how to love, and how not to hate and retaliate.

Q1. What makes love the great commandment? _____

Q2. What is the difference between loving God and self? __

Q3. How can I love with heart, soul, and mind? _____

Q4. How can I love my neighbors? **See how God loves them**.

Q5. What is the law? _____

We need extraordinary love to overcome spiritual disorders. A little bit of love will not do. God is love, the great Healer. He can heal, we cannot.

Q6. Does the Bible teach to hate neighbors? _____

Q7. How can we bless others? _____

Q8. What good do I to others? _____

Q9. For whom do you pray? _____

Q10. What do the sun and rain teach us? _____

Q11. Why should you not retaliate? _____

Q12. How do you change your hate into love? _____

3.43 Spiritual Fruit

The Bible describes the spiritual life as it contrasts with spiritual disorders (SD1-8). The spiritual life is also called the fruit of the spirit, spiritual gifts, living in the spirit and walking in the spirit. Spiritual disorders are called lusts of the flesh, works of the flesh, and cravings of our sinful nature.

People either have an active spiritual life with spiritual fruit or are dominated by material lusts (SD3) and natural cravings (SD4) that are spiritual disorders (SD1-8). Spiritual life leads to life in the kingdom of God, spiritual disorders lead to fear (SD5) and eternal death.

Paul in Galatians 5:16-25 writes:

"16 This I say then, Walk in the Spirit, and you shall not fulfill the lust of the flesh (SD4)."

"17 For the flesh lusts against the Spirit, and the Spirit against the flesh (SD2): and these are contrary the one to the other: so that you cannot do the things that you would."

"22 But the fruit of the Spirit is love (SD2), joy (SD1), peace (SD5), longsuffering, gentleness, goodness (SD7), faith (SD6) 23 meekness, temperance: against such there is no law."

"24 And they that are Christ's have crucified the flesh (SD3) with the affections and lusts (SD4)."

"25 If we live in the Spirit, let us also walk in the Spirit."

Instructions: Discuss and check your one best answer.

16. Walking in the Spirit means to:

___ be guided by spiritual concerns as outlined in the Bible

___ find all your spiritual guidance wherever you can

___ follow in the footsteps of great teachers

16. The lust of the flesh is:

___ spiritual desires

___ in harmony with the spiritual life

___ contrary to the spiritual life

17. Spiritual disorders help us:

___ recognizing the wrong course of our actions

___ learning how good we are

___ appreciating the kingdom of God

22, 23 The fruit of the Spirit is

___ a spiritual disorder

___ a free gift from Christ to His followers

___ a condition of salvation

22, 23 Write in the number of the spiritual disorder associated with each of the following: love___, joy___, peace___, patience___, kindness___, goodness___, faithfulness___, gentleness___, self-control___.

24. Christians find healing for their spiritual disorders by:

___ avoiding sin

___ accepting by faith Christ as Master

___ following God's law and commandments

157

3.44 Life in the Spirit.

Paul, in the book of Romans Chapter 8, writes about life in the spirit and life contrary to the spirit.

"5 Those who are dominated by the sinful nature think about sinful things (SD2), but those who are controlled by the Holy Spirit think about things that please the Spirit (SD1). 6 So letting your sinful nature control your mind leads to death (SD3). But letting the Spirit control your mind leads to life and peace (SD5). 7 For the sinful nature is always hostile to God (SD3). It never did obey God's laws (SD7), and it never will. 8 That's why those who are still under the control of their sinful nature (SD3) can never please God (SD1)." Rom 8:5-8

"28 And we know that God causes everything to work together for the good of those who love God and are called according to his purpose for them."

"38 And I am convinced that nothing can ever separate us from God's love (SD2). Neither death nor life (SD5), neither angels nor demons(SD7), neither our fears for today nor our worries about tomorrow (SD5)—not even the powers of hell (SD3) can separate us from God's love (SD1)."

"39 No power in the sky above or in the earth below—indeed, nothing in all creation (SD4) will ever be able to separate us from the love of God (SD6) that is revealed in Christ Jesus our Lord." Romans 8:28, 38-39

Discuss and answer the following questions.

Q1. How does our sinful nature show itself? _____

Q2. To what does our sinful nature lead us? A2. **To death.** _

Q3. To what does the Spirit lead us? _____

Q4. What is the relationship between God and sin? _____

Q5. How can we obey God's law? _____

Q6. What does it take to please God? _____

Q7. For whom do things work together for good? _____

Q8. What does "creation" include? _____

Q9. What can separate us from God's love? _____

Q10. How is God's love revealed? _____

Q11. What does it mean to live in the spirit? _____

Q12. How do you taste or experience the love of God? _____

3.45 Peter's Spiritual Taxonomy

There are many formal and informal lists of goodness and evil. Peter presents one of such lists in 2 Peter 1:2-8.

2 "Grace and peace be multiplied unto you through the knowledge of God, and of Jesus our Lord."

"3 According as his divine power hath given unto us all things that pertain unto life and godliness, through the knowledge of him that has called us to glory and virtue (SD1)."

"4 Whereby are given unto us exceeding great and precious promises: that by these ye might be partakers of the divine nature, having **escaped the corruption that is in the world** (SD3) through lust (SD4)."

"5 And beside this, giving all diligence, add to your faith virtue (SD7); and to virtue knowledge; 6 And to knowledge temperance; and to temperance patience (SD6); and to patience godliness (SD5); 7 And to godliness brotherly kindness (SD2); and to brotherly kindness charity (SD2)."

"8 For if these things be in you, and abound, they make you that ye shall neither be barren nor unfruitful in the knowledge of our Lord Jesus Christ (SD1)." 2 Peter:1:2-8

Discuss and answer the following questions.

Q1. How does the knowledge of God multiply peace? _____

Q2. How does the knowledge of God call us to virtue? ____

Q3. By what are we partakers of divine nature? _____

Q4. What will we escape? A4. **Worldly corruption.** _____

Q5. What do we have to add to faith? _____

Q6. What is faith? _____

Q7. How does patience help our spiritual life? _____

Q8. What is the difference between kindness and charity? ___

Q9. What is the result of these characteristics? _____

Q10. How does our knowledge of God affect us? _____

Q11. What is our knowledge of God? _____

3.46 Spiritual Guidelines

Solomon, in Proverbs 6:16-19, lists seven things that God hates: "A proud look (SD2), a lying tongue (SD7), hands that shed innocent blood (SD6), a heart that devised wicked plans (SD3), feet that are swift to running to evil (SD4), a false witness who speaks lies (SD5), and one who sows discord among brothers (SD1)".

The Seven Deadly Sins are usually listed as wrath (SD5), greed (SD3), sloth (SD7), pride (SD2), lust (SD4), envy (SD1), and gluttony. In a way, they too may be considered spiritual disorders.

"The Order of the Divine mind, embodied in the Divine Law, is beautiful. What should a man do but try to reproduce it, as far as possible, in his daily life?" C. S. Lewis, Reflections on the Psalms, p. 59.

The psalmist writes: "Lord, who shall abide in thy tabernacle? Who shall dwell in thy holy hill (SD1)? He that walks uprightly, and works righteousness, and speaks the truth in his heart (SD7). He that backbites not with his tongue, nor doeth evil to his neighbor (SD2), nor takes up a reproach against his neighbor (SD6). In whose eyes a vile person is contemned (SD4); but he honors them that fear the Lord. He that swears to his own hurt, and changes not (SD5). He that puts not out his money to usury (SD3), nor takes reward against the innocent. He that doeth these things shall never be moved." Psalm 15: 1-5.

162

Discuss and answer the following questions.

Q1. How does God hate the seven things? _____

Q2. How can we avoid the seven things? _____

Q3. How does God hate the seven sins? _____

Q4. How can we avoid the seven sins? _____

Q5. What happens when we do not avoid the seven sins? _____

Q6. What is the order of the divine mind? _____

Q7. Where is God's tabernacle? _____

Q8. Is God's tabernacle in his holy hills? _____

Q9. How can we live there? _____

Q10. What summarizes these actions? _____

Q11. What moves one out of the tabernacle? **Our sins**_____

3.47 The Farmer Scatters Seeds

A parable in the Bible contrasts spiritual disorder and spiritual order. Spiritual disorder is wasteful, spiritual order is real and productive in life.

"14 The farmer sows the word."

"15 And these are they *by the way side*, where the word is sown; but when they have heard, Satan cometh immediately, and **takes away the word** (SD1) that was sown in their hearts."

"16 And these are they likewise which are sown *on stony ground*; who, when they have heard the word, immediately receive it with gladness;"

"17 And have *no root in themselves*, and so endure but for a time: afterward, when **affliction** (SD6) or **persecution** (SD5) arises for the word's sake, immediately they are **offended** (SD2)."

"18 And these are they which are *sown among thorns*; such as hear the word,"

"19 And the **cares of this world** (SD4), and the **deceitfulness of riches** (SD3), and the **lusts of other things** entering in, choke the word, and it becomes **unfruitful** (SD7)."

"20 And these are they which are *sown on good ground*; such as hear the word, and receive it,"

"and bring forth fruit, some thirtyfold, some sixty, and some an hundred. Mark 4:14-20."

In this parable told by Jesus there are six symbols:

Q1. The farmer stands for _____

Q2. The seed stands for _____

Q3. The road-side seed stands for _____

Q4. The stony ground seed stands for _____

Q5. The seed among thorns stands for _____

Q6. The seed from good soil stands for _____

Q7. How does the absence of the Word of God produce disorder?

_____

Q8. How does the Word of God produce spiritual order?

_____

Q9. What makes the difference between 30, 60, and 100 fold increase in the Word of God?

A9. The frequency with which we use/share God's Word.

(Note: Consider the above questions, but the answers may be difficult to find. There may not be simple answers to these questions. It may be, that the answer to Q9 is to share the encouraging word 30, 60 or 100 times.)

3.48 How shall we then live? Summary and Conclusion

We seem to get into trouble quite naturally. When we are young, we often feel strong and able to do anything. Sickness and death seem far away. It seems impossible that a mental disorder like depression could cloud over all we do. And the spiritual seems like an option that we can ignore.

With time, reality becomes a good teacher. That is, if we let it teach us. We can learn a healthy lifestyle that reduces our chances of physical diseases. Many are able to use their minds wisely and stay out of mental disorders. The big challenge is our spiritual life.

You can do a few things as you follow up on what you explored in this volume.

1. Consider participating in the Klimes Institute Spiritual Disorder Study Conference usually held on the first Monday and Tuesday of October in Sacramento, CA.

2. Contact the Klimes Institute with your suggestions and questions via rudy@klimes.org.

3. Explore some of the 10 books by Dr. Klimes available from online bookstores.

4. Study the websites cecourses.org, conted.org, ethice.org, bibled.org, and klimes.org that are related to the Klimes Institute.

Appendix

Appendix A: Cases of Spiritual Disorder

Below is a list of ten cases, some of which describe a specific spiritual disorder and some do not. Place the number of the disorder in front of the cases that describe a specific disorder.

a. ____ Joe is somewhat overactive at work, home and play.

b. ____ Mary has a good appetite but is not gaining weight.

c. ____ Bill has stopped reading books and following the news.

d. ____ Ted loves his little garden and keeps planting flowers.

e. ____ Jane regularly attends her Bible Study group.

f. ____ Mike has given up hope of ever finding a good job.

g. ____ Joan is planning her family reunion.

h. ____ Frank weekly cuts his old neighbor's grass.

i. ____ Ron has difficulty sleeping, and getting a good night's rest.

j. ____ John feels tired much of the time.

Appendix B: Educational Lesson Plan and FAITH

a. Title:

b. Objectives:

c. Topics to Teach:

d. Materials:

e. Step-By-Step Procedures:

f. Plan for Independent Practice:

g. Assessment Based on Objectives:

King, D. E. (2002). **Spirituality and Medicine. FAITH**. <http://www.pastoraljournal.findaus.com/pdfs/ar2.pdf>

F – Do you have a **Faith** or religion that is important to you?

A – How do your beliefs **Apply** to your health?

I – Are you **Involved** in a church or faith community?

T – How do your spiritual views affect your views about **Treatment?**

H – How can I **Help** you with any spiritual concerns?

Appendix C: Basic Spiritual Interventions

Initials _____ Date _____ Phone_____

After diagnosis, check one or more of the below blanks.

___1. Intentional Ministry of Presence

___2. Meaning Making

___3. Grief Work

___4. Clinical Use of Prayer

___5. Confession – Guilt

___6. Forgiveness Work

___7. Thanking

___8. Life Review – Spiritual Autobiography

___9. Scripture Education

___10. Reframing God Assumptions

___11. Encouraging Connection with a Spiritual Community

___12. Creative Writing

___13. No Intervention needed

Appendix D: Spiritual Diagnostic Worksheet:

Initials _____Date _____Phone_____

After diagnosis, check one or more of the below blanks:

____2.1 Joylessness Disorder: __Mild, __Moderate, __Severe

____2.2 Self-centeredness Disorder: Mild, _Moderate, Severe

____2.3 Materialistic Disorder: __Mild, __Moderate, __Severe

____2.4 Pleasure-seeking Disorder: Mild, __Moderate,_Severe

____2.5 Fear Disorder: __Mild, __Moderate, __Severe

____2.6 Unforgiving Disorder: __Mild, _Moderate, ___Severe

____2.7 Dishonesty Disorder: __Mild, __Moderate, __Severe

____2.8 Unspecified Disorder: __Mild, __Moderate, __Severe

Diagnosed as _____

____3.0 No Disorder

Appendix E: A Plan for Developing Self-Control

Spiritual Disorders can be healed by the exercise of self-control. The plan below is provided as a free public service by the Bridge Resource Centre.

"1. Admit my lack of discipline. I don't understand what I do: for I don't do what I would like to, but instead I do what I hate! For even though the desire to do good is in me, I'm not able to do it." Romans 7:15, 18 (GN)

"2. Believe that God will help me. For it is God who works in you to will and do what pleases Him." Philippians 2:13 (NLT)

"3. Claim a promise from the Bible. Do not fear, for I am with you; do not be dismayed, for I am your God. I will strengthen you and help you." Isaiah 41:10 (NLT) "God has not given us the spirit of fear, but the spirit of power and of love and of self-discipline (self-control)." 2 Timothy 1:7 (NLT) "I can do all things through Christ who strengthens me. Philippians 4:13."

"4. Decide in advance." Proverbs 13:16 (NIV)

"5. Tell a friend. Two are better than one because if one falls down, the other can help him up. Two can resist an attack that would defeat one man alone." Ecclesiastes 4:9-10, 12 (GN)

"6. Focus on the reward. Self-control is delayed gratification. It is postponing pleasure in order to fulfill a greater purpose."

Appendix F: Seven Spiritual Health Problem Areas

Seven general spiritual health problem areas affect all or most spiritual disorders. The seven pointers are provided by Brian Childs and Pam Moss as a public service at the Bridge Family Resource Centre. < http://www.okbridgefamilies.com/>

"1. UNCLEAR PURPOSE: I have labored to no purpose; I have spent my strength in vain and for nothing." Isaiah 49:4

"2. UNEMPLOYED TALENT: Each should live his life with the gifts the Lord has given him ..." 1 Corinthians 7:17

"3. UNBALANCED SCHEDULE: Take the time and the trouble to keep yourself spiritually fit." 1 Timothy 4:7b

"4. UNCONFESSED SIN: My guilt has overwhelmed me like a burden too heavy to bear...I am bowed down." Psalm 38:4-6

"5. UNRESOLVED CONFLICT: Resentment destroys the fool, and jealousy kills the simple." Job 5:2. "You are only hurting yourself with your anger." Job 18:4

"6. UNSUPPORTED LIFESTYLE: Two are better than one, if one falls down, his friend can help him up. But pity the man who falls and has no one to help him up." Ecclesiastes 4:9-10

"7. UNDERNOURISHED SPIRIT: Let your roots grow down into Him and draw up nourishment from Him. See that you go on growing in the Lord, and become strong." Colossians 2:6-7"

SUMMARY: To diagnose physical diseases, physicians us the International Classification of Diseases (ICD). To diagnose mental disorders, psychiatrists and psychologists use the Diagnostic and Statistical Manuel of Mental Disorders (DSM). Up to now, chaplains and pastors had no broadly-based classification to diagnose spiritual disorders.

The mission of this present volume is to fill this need and to provide a classification of spiritual disorders. It is expected that this volume will go through a number of revisions before it reaches its optimal usefulness. To find help with Spiritual Disorders, healing of each of the eight disorders is examined from a research, ethics and faith perspective.

A Word of Thanks

A small group of health professionals has assisted in this effort and has made needed suggestions. They are Paul Kramer, MD; Chaplain Tim Thompson, DMin; Sharon Perry, RN Nurse Practitioner; Lian Funada, RN, BSN, PHN; Howard Munson, DDS; Pastor Eddie Heinrich, DMin; Joyce Knight-Bennett, EdD, educator; Anna Klimes, EdD, retired professor; Bonnie Klimes-Dougan, PhD, assistant professor; Pastor James Campbell, MA; and John Raphael, MSc. Engineer. Their assistance has been much appreciated.

About the Author

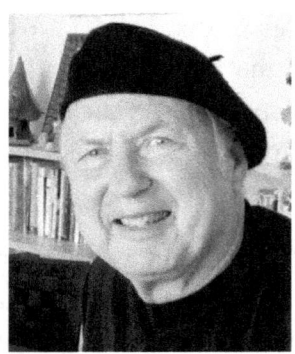

Rudolf Klimes was born in Czechoslovakia. The son of a Jew, he survived Hitler's holocaust and escaped Stalin's Iron Curtain. He served as college president in Korea, Japan, and Hong Kong. Klimes received his BA and MA in 1957 from Walla Walla University and his EdS and PhD in 1964 from Indiana University. In 1977, he earned a MA at Andrews University, in 1981 a DMin at McCormick Theological Seminary, and in 1983 a MPH at Johns Hopkins University.

From 1973 to 1979, he directed the Graduate Programs in Educational Administration at Andrews University, Michigan. He wrote some 30 research reports and ten books.

In 1979, he was elected Associate Director of the General Conference Health Department in Washington, DC. In 1986, he returned to Asia as president of Samyuk College in Hong Kong, and from 1989 to1995 served as founding Dean of Lifelong Learning at Sahmyook University, in Korea. Since 1995, Anna and he live and serve in the Sacramento area.

174

References

Aristotle. (350 BC). Rhetoric II:7. Translated by Edghill, E. M. Retrieved from http://classics.mit.edu/Aristotle/categories.html.

Aristotle. (350 BC). Nicomachean Ethics, Translated by Edghill, E. M. I-8. Retrieved from http://classics.mit.edu/Aristotle/categories.html.

Bekelman, David B., Sydney, M., Dy, M. Diane M. Becker, Wittstein, Ilan S., Hendricks, Danetta E., Yamashita, Traci E., & Gottlieb Sheldon H. (2007, April). Spiritual Well-Being and Depression in Patients with Heart Failure. *J Gen Intern Med. 22(4):* 470–477.

Berridge, Kent, C., & Kringelbach, Morten L. (2011, October 12). Building a neuroscience of pleasure and well-being. *Psychol Well Being. 1(1):* 1–3.

Boscarino, Joseph, Adams, E Richard, Figley Charles R., Galea, Sanro, & Foa Edna B. (2009 June 23). Fear of Terrorism and Preparedness in New York City 2 Years After the Attacks: Implications for Disaster Planning and Research. *J Public Health Manag Pract. PMC.*

Card, Orson, Scott, San Angelo, Letters to an Incipient Heretic, Speaker for the Dead. Retrieved from www.orsonscottcard.com.

Chang, Maria Hsia. (2009). Pathological Narcissism, A Spiritual Disorder. Professor, Political Science, University of Nevada, Reno. Retrieved from http://abusesanctuary.blogspot.com/2007/02/pathological-narcissism-spiritual.html .

Cicirelli, Victor G., Gerontol J. (2009, January). Sibling Death and Death Fear in Relation to Depressive Symptomatology in Older Adults. Sci *Soc Sci. 64B(1):* 24–32.

Diagnostic and Statistical Manuel of Mental Disorders, IV Edition (DSM-IV). (2000). American Psychiatric Association, Arlington, VA.

Föller-Mancini, Axel, Heusser Peter, & Büssing, Arndt. (2010). Self-centeredness in Adolescents: An empirical study of students of Steiner schools, Christian academic high schools, and public schools. *Research on Steiner Education,* Vol. 1 No 2.

Frances, Allen. (2009, October). A Warning Sign on the Road to DSM-V: Beware of Its Unintended Consequences. *UBM Medica Psychiatric Times.*

Greenberger, Dennis, & Padesky, Christine. (1995). Mind Over Mood: Change How You Feel by Changing the Way You Think. *(The Guilford Press,* New York*).*

Harris, Alex H. S. & Thorsen, Carl E. (2005). Forgiveness, Unforgiveness, Health, and Disease. Retrieved   from

http://www.chce.research.va.gov/docs/pdfs/pi_publicatio
ns/Harris/2005_Harris_Thorsen_HF.pdf .

Hodge, D. R., Horvath, & V. E. (2011, October). Spiritual
Needs in Health Care Settings: a Qualitative Meta-synthesis
of Clients' Perspectives. *Social Work*. *56(4):*306-16.

Hodge, S. R. (1949, October). Men, Machines, and
Materialism, *Br Med J*.

Hospice and Palliative Nursing Association. (2008). Signs and
Symptoms of Spiritual Distress.

Hummel, Leonard et al. Spiritual Categories of Intervention.
(2008). *Journal of Health Care Chaplaincy* 15:40-51.

Kalish, N. (2012, June). Evidence-based Spiritual Care: a
Literature Review. *Current Opinion Supporting Palliative
Care. 6(2):*242-6.

King, D. E. (2002). Spirituality and Medicine. FAITH.
Retrieved   from
http://www.pastoraljournal.findaus.com/pdfs/ar2.pdf.

Ku Ya Lie. (2007). Ku Spiritual Distress Scale. Fooyin
University of Taiwan.

Lewis, C. S. (1964). Reflections on the Psalms, Mariner
Books: Seattle. 59.

Maselko, J, S., Gilman, E., & Buka, S. (2009, June) Religious service attendance and spiritual well-being are differentially associated with risk of major depression. *Psychol Med. 39(6):* 1009–1017.

Mead, Nicole L., Baumeister F., Gino, Francesca, Schweitzer,Maurixe E., & Ariely Dan. (2009). Too Tired to Tell the Truth: Self-Control Resource Depletion and Dishonesty. *J Exp Soc Psychol. 45(3):* 594–597.

Monod, Stefanie, Rochat, Etienne, Christophe J Büla, Guy Jobin, Estelle Martin, & Brenda Spencer. (2010). The spiritual distress assessment tool: an instrument to assess spiritual distress in hospitalized elderly persons. *BMC Geriatr.* 10: 88.

Monod, S, Brennan, M., Rochat E., Martin E, Rochat S, & Büla C. J. (2011, November). Instruments measuring spirituality in clinical research: a systematic review. *J Gen Intern Med. 26 (11):* 1345-57.

Moreland, J.P. (1997). Love your God with all your mind: The role of reason in the life of the soul. *Colorado Springs, CO. Navpress Publishing Co.*

Northridge, W. L. (1961). Disorders of the Emotional and Spiritual Life, Great Neck, NY: Channel Press.

Puchalski, C. M., Kilpatrick, S. D., McCullough, M. E., & Larson, D. B. (2003, March). A systematic review of spiritual and religious variables in Palliative Medicine, American Journal of Hospice and Palliative Care, Hospice Journal,

Journal of Palliative Care, and Journal of Pain and Symptom Management. *Palliative Support Care. 1(1):*7-13.

Sip, Kamila E., Skewes, Joshua C., Marchant, Jennifer. L., McGregor, William B., Roepstorff, Andreas, & Frith, Christopher D. (2012). What if I Get Busted? Deception, Choice, and Decision-Making in Social Interaction. *Front Neurosci.* 6: 58.

Smith, David B. (2007, May 15). Addiction as a Spiritual Disease, *Articlesbase*, Retrieved from www.articlesbase.com/religion-articles/addiction-as-a-spiritual-disease-147644.html.

Talwar, Victoria, Gordon, Lee, Heidi, & Kang M. (2007, May). Lying in the Elementary School Years. *Dev Psychol. 43(3):* 804–810.

Touro Institute, Spiritual Assessment and Care, Retrieved December 2012 from http://www.touroinstitute.com/6%20Spiritual%20Assessment%20and%20Care.pdf.

Trollope, Anthony. Autobiography of Anthony Trollope. Retrieved October 2012 from www.anthonytrollope.com.

Verghese, Abraham. (2008, October-December). Spirituality and mental health. *Indian J Psychiatry. 50(4):* 233–237.

Whybrow, Peter. (2005). American Mania: When More Is Not Enough. *MedGenMed*. 7(3): 70. Reviewed by Hayes Virginia M. and Zylowska Lidia.

Yong J, Kim J, Han S.S, & Puchalski C.M. (2008, Winter). Development and validation of a scale assessing spiritual needs for Korean patients with cancer. *J Palliat Care. 24(4):*240-6.

Notes

National Library of Medicine. (Information that is created by or for the US government on this site is within the public domain. Public domain information on the National Library of Medicine (NLM) Web pages may be freely distributed and copied. www.ncbi.nlm.nih.gov/pmc/articles). This covers the research journal articles quoted.

The volume documentation follows in general the American Psychological Association (APA) style of documentation, 6th edition. Where research journal abstracts are given, they are usually presented as titles before rather than after the quotations, and the title itself is presented in bold type.